SONG FOR THE AGING MALE

Throwing off the shackles of youth,
I reached for the stars!
…And pulled a hip flexor.

Dammit.

CONTENTS

PROLOGUE

A Medical Centrist's Prescription for the Aging Middle-Aged Guy

Look at you! Your soul patch has migrated to your earlobes. Anything larger than a saltine after 8:00 p.m. gives you heartburn deep into the twilight hours. Emptying your bladder is no longer like one of those snappy station breaks on TV, but more like a 60-second commercial complete with a celebrity spokesperson and theme music. A bad night of sleep makes you feel like you just finished an Ironman triathlon. For heaven's sake, you tore your Achilles tendon just walking the dog.

It was fun while it lasted: youth, that magical, ethereal out-of-body experience, a kind of natural hallucinogenic state in which the world smiles at us. One's healthy, vigorous, capable body is almost an afterthought, a perfectly engineered machine that seems unfazed by bad food habits, missed sleep, or spontaneous feats of exercise.

But eventually that youthful you—so maintenance free, so under the radar, so unappreciated—starts to change. The celestial body you inhabited back in your twenties is now returning squarely to Earth, and you have to admit that although the gravitational pull of time can be resisted, it cannot be rebuffed.

At some point you realize you've gone from MC Hammer's "U Can't Touch This" to Time Warner's Smokin' Oldies collection called *Don't Touch That. It Hurts When You Touch That. My Back Is on Fire. Where Is My Heating Pad?* You busted a move, all right, and your doc says it'll take six to eight weeks to heal.

And that, as we like to say in the medical world, sucks. Getting older is an extractive, reductive process, and given its relentless and inevitable nature, it might be the hardest thing any of us will ever do.

If you're lucky, this won't be a solo expedition to the far reaches of Geezerville. You'll have a partner along for the ride. In fact, there's a good chance that your partner is behind the wheel, reading this book for you, taking some ownership of your body and health in a blatant act of benevolent theft. Bravo!

Man Overboard! aims to help you get through this pilgrimage to Geezerville, this magical journey of aging-while-male, not unscathed but with a sense of control and dignity. You can get more of both of those if you understand how your body works, what happens when it doesn't, and how to fix it. Separating social media hearsay, manipulative Big Pharma marketing schemes, and "old husbands' tales" from the truth won't lower your cholesterol, but it will give you some clarity.

What you'll discover in the following pages is that I am a medical centrist. That's because, generally speaking, the truth lies somewhere in the middle. You don't want high blood pressure, but you don't want low blood pressure, either. Right in the middle is good. You want a strong heart, but if it gets too muscular, it gets stiff and then it doesn't work right. Thyroid function? Middle, please. Too much and you get wired up like a meth addict without the dental issues. Too little and you start to feel cold, slow, and pudgy.

On one extreme of personal health, you have the neurotically health-obsessed. Every facet of life, every food choice, every moment of activity, every guilty pleasure is either adding to or removing seconds from life. Every symptom must be pursued as a warning sign that will allow them to take action. But every piece of health information can also be perceived as just one more way to die, and these people often end up worried sick—sometimes literally. Sure, it's possible that all that effort will allow them to live longer, but how much longer, and will they even enjoy it?

On the other extreme of personal health is just straight-up denial, sometimes referred to as "testosterone blindness" or "testosterone poisoning." Equal parts stoicism, nihilism, and good old-fashioned fear, this is the feeling that a guy can be completely healthy as long as he doesn't go to the doctor, who might "give" him diabetes, high blood pressure, or prostate cancer. "I was perfectly fine when I walked in the clinic door!" But "I am fine, because I have been fine, and so I will continue to be fine" is not a legitimate medical self-evaluation, and delaying care generally just leads to bigger problems.

I get it. I hate going to the doctor, too. I treat shopping and health care like a special-ops mission: a high-risk venture pursued only out of great necessity and with a sense of urgency. You get in there, get what you need, and get the hell out! If I could get a chopper to extricate me, I would (extraction point: Cinnabon, upper level of food court).

One might think aging would be easier for a doctor—so much inside knowledge—but all that does is make us the world's most well-informed hypochondriacs. Pinning the diagnosis tail on the symptoms donkey is what I do for a living, and it comes too easily. For example, as I, the doctor, quite rationally tell myself that the most plausible explanation for the ringing in my left ear is last weekend's high-decibel concert, my doctor's mind also considers the distinctly unlikely and yet *very real* possibility of a brain tumor called an "acoustic neuroma." That same brain imagines the local headlines: VILLAGE IDIOT DOCTOR IGNORES OBVIOUS BRAIN TUMOR SYMPTOMS. Being an aging doctor isn't easy, and in some ways, I've written this book for myself—me, the aging middle-aged guy.

Man Overboard! is a middle ground for the midlife health crisis. Think of it like investing in the stock market: you want to be involved, and you need to be smart about it, but you don't want to obsess (we all know someone whose mood swings daily with the Dow Jones average), and you don't want to outsmart yourself (overactive trading is a strong predictor of poor performance). You can't outguess the Market, but you can develop a plan that gives you the best chance of having a healthy financial future.

It's the same with your personal health: you want to take control of your health without being out of control. You want a plan—a rational plan—and then you want to get on with your life. And a key part of that plan is understanding your health risks, so that you can make the most important things the most important things.

As I write, coronavirus is taking a no-expenses-paid trip around the world. Hospitals are becoming overwhelmed, and the global economy's sweater is unraveling. In the United States, COVID deaths have surpassed the number of US military killed in the Vietnam conflict, and it's unclear how much fuel the loosening of social restrictions will add to the pandemic fire.

For most of April, 2020 COVID-19 was jockeying back and forth with heart disease and cancer for the daily leading cause of death in the United States, but coronavirus will eventually fade as immunity, via vaccination or actual infection, rises. And whatever the "new normal" turns out to be, cancer and heart disease will almost certainly remain atop the leaderboard for the most common causes of death. So let's get those two right. Let's make sure we understand the diseases, the risk factors, the screening tests—information that is concise enough to remember, and clear enough to act on. Conversely, although *Man Overboard!* will give you a lot of information on something as common and consequential as heart disease, it will skip over coronavirus, shark attacks, jousting-related deaths, and the like.

We'll start with maladies that matter but don't immediately pose a lethal threat: "I'm losing my edge, I can't get it up, I'm going bald, my back hurts, I can't quit smoking, I can't sleep, I need to eat better and exercise more, I'm getting a little pudgy. Or, let's be honest: I'm sporting the Jim Gaffigan marshmallow abs." These are things we all deal with, and even though they don't hit like heart attacks, how we manage the little stuff, including making little lifestyle changes that add up to big health benefits, informs how likely we are to get the big stuff right. Like the hairball you pulled out of the shower drain, everything is connected.

A couple more things before we dispense with this seemingly endless preview and get on with our show.

First, *Man Overboard!* is for every man—regardless of skin color, nationality, sexual orientation, culture, body shape/BMI, hair pattern, shoe size, or IPA preference. The national reckoning we are experiencing over the enduring effects of systemic racism also extends into the medical field, where modern medicine and genetics are reminding us all that race is a social construct, not a biological one. Ironically, humans chose one obvious but *nearly inconsequential* genetic difference—the amount of melanin pigment in our skin—to separate us into different groups that were then shamefully assigned *highly consequential* social implications. We could have chosen to exploit any such minor difference: head shape, left- or right-handedness, eye color, or even ear wax composition (seriously, there are two genetically distinct kinds of ear wax). But the nod went to skin color. It turns out that the owner's manual for Homo sapiens contains very few asterisks. Most of the health outcomes attributed to race were either due to culture-related health behaviors (dietary habits, for instance) or so-called social determinants of health: poverty, lack of access to healthy food, health care, etc. We are remarkably the same on the inside. And so the words inside *Man Overboard!* are for every man.

Next, I have the audacious goal of making *Man Overboard!* an entertaining read. Most health books are like a colonoscopy: sure, they give you plenty of medical information, but that doesn't make them any easier to sit through. Staying healthy is serious business, but all of us have what I call a "seriousness quotient," and when it's exceeded, one feels either fearful, uninterested, snoozy, or all of those things. So we'll take some mental breaks, and I'll go on a tangent here and there, and then we'll get back to business.

A disclaimer: This book isn't trying to sell you anything (there are many books that are, and some of them are written by doctors). And if you're looking for an encyclopedic book on health, this ain't it. The Internet can be that for you, but if you're not a great swimmer, a deeper pool just gives you more water to drown in.

So, beware and be wary. Fight what you can; surrender to what you must. No doubt about it—life saves the hardest part for last, and given how the odds are stacked, you'll do better with an open hand rather than a closed fist.

Be informed. Embrace change, but have a healthy skepticism about the Next Big Thing in health care. Like the marble you swallowed as a kid, it will eventually pass. And keep in mind that a sense of humor and low expectations can get you through anything, except Customs and a really bad marriage. As Kentucky farmer, writer, poet, and Master of the Universe Wendell Berry has written in his book *The Mad Farmer Poems*:

> *Laughter is immeasurable. Be joyful*
> *though you have considered all the facts.*

There must be some dignified way to get through all of this. Text me if you find it.

I hope you enjoy this book.

Craig Bowron, M.D.
Saint Paul, Minnesota

What goes around comes up
on back of you,
because the globe is roundish.
It's not perfectly round—like an egg—
but more like a racquetball.

—*Miracle Nutrition with Hearty White*

ANDROPAUSE

The "Age of Getting Things Done" Begs the Shadowy Question, "Is It Low T?"

When it comes to the hormonal changes of growing older, women get the message on a billboard called "menopause." They get hot flashes that have the geothermic intensity of a solar flare; one can hear the air conditioner groan as it tries to keep up. The uterus sputters and coughs and smokes like an old lawn mower engine. And so they go to book groups and coffee shops to commiserate; they support each other with kindly, upbeat text messages as they go through their Great Change.

Men get the message on a small post-card, or rather a series of small postcards, the first of which states, "It's a small injury, but it'll take weeks to recover." Many of these postcards arrive in the morning, when you arise to some new pain and ask yourself, "What did I do to make it feel this way?" And then later on that morning you'll realize it's because yesterday you hauled three cases of soda out of the car to a nearby picnic pavilion. How pathetic— three cases of soda!

MAN OVERBOARD!

THIS IS THE AGE of getting things done with silly ED ads. Unclear what "Low T" really is, either by symptoms or even lab testing, and whether it is safe to replace it without increasing the risk of prostate cancer or heart disease. Proceed with caution.

Crippled by a lifetime of testosterone poisoning, we simply ignore our demise; or, failing that, we keep it to ourselves. There is a strength and nobility—and also dysfunction and suffering—in going it alone, and we gladly bear the load.

Dear Craig,
weather is here,
wish you were
beautiful!
Good luck in the
shadows!
— Andropause

TO:

If, just hypothetically speaking, there were an "andropause"—a more subtle, nebulous version of "womenopause"—how would one find out more information about it? From the marketing professionals of Big Pharma, of course! The development of erectile dysfunction drugs in the late '90s, Androgel's FDA approval in 2000, and Solvay Pharmaceuticals 2008 launch of the "Low T"/Androgel campaign ushered in a golden era of marketing that "clarified" for us and for television viewers what andropause looked like.

Big Pharma spent big money bringing the erectile dysfunction (ED) message to the public with direct-to-consumer advertising. In 2008, for example, they shelled out over $300 million hawking ED drugs, a figure that put them atop the direct-to-consumer leaderboard and out-paced advertising on drugs for osteoporosis, insomnia, auto-immune disorders (rheumatoid arthritis, etc.), and heart disease. Ad money goes where the money is, not necessarily where the greatest health need is.

Unfortunately, this heady epoch when Pecker Power drugs and testosterone gels ruled the television world began to fizzle out in 2017 when Pfizer reached a settlement with Teva Pharmaceuticals to allow them to produce a generic version of Viagra (a generic had been available in Europe since 2013). When generics show up, branded drugs experience icewater–like sales shrinkage—as much as 90 percent. Still, like the wisdom of an ancient text, the message of these ads continues to speak to aging males, particularly those who enjoy being satirized.

Commercializing the Paradox of the Aging Male: Strong but Weak, Old but Young, Impotent but Lusty...

In all fairness, these marketeers had a difficult task before them. They needed to present the image of a strong man who the consumer would want to emulate, while also presenting a protagonist who was wounded—deeply, but not in any deeply obvious way. A man who was virile and yet impotent. A man who was cocksure and yet depressed. A man who was recognizably older but not *old*—and no paunch! And how ironic that is, given the fact that obesity is the leading cause of adult diabetes, one of the main risk factors for erectile dysfunction. In other words, they left the poster child for ED off the poster.

Our poster boy should have thick, luxurious hair but with graying temples. He hasn't lost *it*—his hair or his machismo—yet, or at least not permanently. Finally, he should be a take-charge kind of guy. Whether it's hauling two clawfoot bathtubs to the edge of the ocean surf, or organizing a blues band with his buddies in a desert roadhouse, the maturing male is a doer, capable of acting out even the most thinly veiled sexual metaphors ("Can I still throw the ol' pigskin through that tire swing?").

Speaking of titillating metaphors, there's the Viagra motto, "This is the age of getting things done." Who doesn't enjoy "doing it"? You get this done by doing someone. If you do it, then you're done—you did it, and then you did it again, and then it was done. That's how you do it. Other variations of the motto included, "This is the age of knowing how to make things happen," and "of taking action," but those don't do it for me. Although I do like to do it. I like to get things done.

...and also, Stupid but Resourceful

Perhaps the most enjoyable aspect of these ads was how bungling and dimwitted the gray-templed protagonist could look. A cattle rancher is pulling a horse trailer through a wide-open, wind-scarred valley in Montana. The problem—a gigantic mud puddle, alias erectile dysfunction—is right in the middle of the road. And though he could easily have driven around it, the dumbass drives right into her and gets stuck up to the hubs. At which point he backs out his team of horses (alias Viagra) from the trailer and pulls the truck free.

In a Camaro ad, the guy pulls into an archetypal vintage desert gas station with a steaming radiator. He ambles inside, grabs a bottle of mineral water from the cooler, saunters back outside, takes a swig for himself, and then pours the rest into the steaming radiator. The viewer doesn't know how he got the radiator cap off, but if he did it with his hands, when the radiator was hot, he could have easily given himself a steam bath that would have put him in the Radiator Springs burn unit. And pouring cold water in a hot engine block runs the risk of cracking it. From the look of it, this is the age of getting things *dumb*.

This Is the Age of Stepping Into the Shadows. "Help! Where Am I?! Who Dimmed the Lights?"

Maybe I was watching too hard, but the ED ads had me worried about andropause. Would I recognize the symptoms, and if so, could I handle them?

Fortunately for me and millions of others, by 2012 the new owner of Androgel, Abbott Laboratories, had its "Is it LowT?" campaign in high gear, flooding the airwaves with educational images of what andropause might look like. One of the TV spots from early in the campaign featured a pudgy, graying, middle-aged male pining for more energy and passion for his favorite pursuits: golf, sex, family, and friends, in that order. A basketball-themed ad included the oddly phrased question, "Don't have the hots for hoops with your buddies?"

The message to men was clear: it's okay to put sports atop your hierarchy of needs, and it would be a mistake to blame your dwindling hots for hoops and fizzling short irons game solely on getting older. The ads counseled viewers to "stop living in the shadows," an ironic slogan choice given how shadowy the science of testosterone in the aging male is.

The fog rolled in as soon as viewers took the Low T Quiz offered on Abbott's "Is It Low T?" website. The quiz consisted of 10 symptom-based questions, many of them vague and entertaining, such as,

"Are you falling asleep after dinner?" or, "Do you have a decrease in strength and/or endurance?" The quiz seemed more like something dreamed up by the Cartoon Network, but it was actually developed by a group of physicians in St. Louis and then borrowed by Abbott.

The problem isn't the questions or who came up with them. The problem is that the symptoms of low testosterone and natural aging are remarkably similar, so that even a smartly developed screening tool is not very discriminating. Asking an aging man (or an aging woman, for that matter) question #2, "Do you have a lack of energy?" is like asking fish if they sometimes suffer from a sense of moistness. My favorite question has to be #8: "Have you noticed a recent deterioration in your ability to play sports?" As a 57-year-old, Family Dollar store–sponsored athlete, I can answer with a firm "no." I have seen a *progressive* deterioration in my athletic abilities since my early 30s, thank you very much.

There are a couple of more pointed questions in the Low T Quiz, such as "Are your erections less strong?" and "Do you have a decrease in libido (sex drive)?" but as incriminating as those might sound, they still don't reveal much about the quiz-taker's testosterone level.

Using data from the long-running European Male Ageing Study, researchers tried to delineate what symptoms most strongly correlated with low testosterone levels. They concluded, "The prevalence of even the most specific sexual symptoms of androgen [testosterone] deficiency was relatively high among men with unequivocally normal testosterone levels." Although an erection may seem to be the pinnacle effect of testosterone, the feat is more physiologic than hormonal; the majority of men with erectile dysfunction have *normal* testosterone levels but *abnormal* circulation or nerve function.

Is It TTT—Time to Test Testosterone Levels?

If taking the Low T Quiz gives you performance anxiety, then it's off to the doctor for something far more objective and exacting than ubiquitous symptoms: a testosterone level. Over a lifespan, testosterone levels reach a peak in our late 20's or early 30's and then drop 1-2 percent a year. On a daily basis, testosterone levels fluctuate a bit, generally peaking around 8 a.m. and then falling by about 30% to a trough around 8 p.m.

Beyond those simple facts is where the shadows deepen. Blood pressure norms have been standardized—less than 120/80 is what we doctors would loosely call "normal." But testosterone levels have a lot of individual variation: normal range is between 250 and 900, depending on the lab that performs the test. The fact that two individuals can have a 200 percent difference in their testosterone levels but have similar libido, muscle function, etc. demonstrates just how crude the measure is.

A test called a "free testosterone level" is perhaps a more accurate physiological indicator of what is going on inside the body, but it's hardly clairvoyant. And whether we're checking total testosterone or free testosterone, should we hold a 75-year-old man to the same standard as a 45-year-old, or should the "normal" levels be pared down in an age-dependent manner? Currently we hold them to the same standard, but the question raises a central debate: are low testosterone levels a "mistake"—a complication of aging that should be treated? Or are they intentional, a genetically programmed adjustment that we should not tamper with?

We grappled with this idea in menopausal women, and spent years strongly encouraging, maybe even *nagging* them, to shore up their sagging hormone levels by starting "HRT"—hormone replacement therapy. Unfortunately, data from the Women's Health Initiative, a powerful study that followed a large number of women for a very long time, eventually showed that HRT increased the risk of heart disease, stroke, and breast cancer. Whoops.

The bulk of the studies on testosterone therapy have been the opposite of that: small numbers of participants, followed for very short periods of time. That might be why, in 2004, the prestigious Institute of Medicine (IOM) completed a systematic review of the medical literature on testosterone therapy trials in older men and found no clear evidence of benefit for any of the health outcomes examined, and that includes machismo. They particularly focused on placebo-controlled trials, which are critically important in a therapy targeted at reducing subjective symptoms (energy, libido) rather than objective findings (e.g., blood pressure).

From the IOM findings came the impetus for the Testosterone Trials, a large, multicenter trial sponsored by the National Institutes of Health and the National Institute on Aging. The T Trials looked to see if testosterone replacement therapy for those with low T could help in seven particular areas. Here's what they found:

1. Sexual function: moderate improvement, more in libido than erections
2. Physical function: small increase in six-minute walking distance
3. Vitality: no change in energy level, but mood a little better
4. Anemia (red blood cells): yes, anemia improved
5. Bones: increased density and strength
6. Cardiovascular: increased atherosclerosis in coronary arteries
7. Cognitive function: can you repeat the question? No, it didn't help.

Many were hoping that the results of the T Trials would answer all of our questions, but they didn't.

The participants were a mean age of 72, which leaves out a lot of middle-aged men, and many not-so-middle-aged men. To qualify for the trial, one had to have a testosterone level that was clearly low, lower than 275 (normal is 250 to 900). Interestingly, only about 15 percent of men who applied for the trial met that criteria, proving yet again the flimsy relationship between presumptive *symptoms* of low T and *actual* low T levels. And the trial lasted only a year, which is long enough to measure a potential benefit, but not long enough to really assess the most concerning risks: accelerated coronary disease and increased risk of prostate cancer. Remember, prostate cancer needs androgen stimulation, which is why starving it of testosterone is a treatment option.

Since the results of the T Trials were released starting in 2016, little has changed. In 2020, the American College of Physicians performed a sweeping review of the risks and benefits of testosterone treatment for men with age-related low testosterone. They made a somewhat lukewarm recommendation for using it to improve sexual dysfunction, noting that physicians should first discuss benefits and possible harms with the patient, and if started, re-evaluate in a year. The expert panel did not recommend that testosterone treatment be used to improve energy, vitality, physical function, or cognition. Of note: they found that testosterone therapy caused either a small or no increase in cardiovascular events, but the evidence was weak.

Is Aging a Natural Process, Not to Be Tampered With? Because If It Ain't Broken, It'll Be Hard to Fix

Okay ladies, we admit it: andropause isn't the BASE jumping hormonal free fall that womenopause is for you. But the concerns about unintended consequences of our testosterone therapy are just as real as the ones for your version of hormone replacement therapy.

So the riddle continues: are some parts of growing older truly pathologic, a disease in need of fixing? Or are there seasons of life, and the deer-camo muscle tee (the one she quietly despises, I might add) that you wore aaallllllll last summer may not work for you in the dark of winter. Hormones that are so pivotal to our younger selves may well have entirely different ramifications as we age. Going deaf to the song of testosterone might be a way in which older, aging tissues protect themselves.

Let's take a drive through an aqua-blue desert in a Camaro SS and figure this all out. And this time, let's bring radiator fluid and a pair of gloves.

2 TESTOSTERONE TALES

The Transformative Powers of the Y Chromosome, and the Complex World of Sex Hormones

Chemically speaking, the difference between the estrogen and testosterone molecules is like the difference between "intimate apparel" and "imminent peril." The two sound very similar, but in the end they're quite different.

You don't have to have a degree in chemistry to follow this: to go from testosterone to estrogen, all you have to do is lop off a methyl group (CH_3) and add a hydrogen (H). Try it yourself. It's not that hard.

This chemical switcheroo is performed by the enzyme aromatase. Although the subtle alteration doesn't seem like much, it's at least a partial explanation for why a young girl cradles her doll with nurturing affection, and a young boy takes the same doll and uses it as a hammer to bludgeon a fleet of attacking droids. Or for the difference between a female singles ad ("I'm looking for an outgoing, caring, intelligent…") and a male singles ad ("Let me tell you about myself…").

But while outward differences between the sexes sometimes seem black and white, from a biochemical perspective, it's much more complicated than that.

Even the "manliest man," whatever

MAN OVERBOARD!

SRY gene gets the ball(s) rolling, and testosterone critical in male development. Yet testosterone and estrogen found in both sexes, albeit in different proportions. Sex hormone levels in the blood are a crude measure—the first signal in a complex cascade of events that happen inside cells, where the hormonal "message" is interpreted and acted on. 'Pink' brain and 'blue' brain far more similar than different, with more inputs than just hormones.

that means, has some estrogen; and even the "girliest girl," whatever that means, has some testosterone.

We still don't understand it all very well, but here's a primer.

In the Beginning, There Was... the SRY Gene
Let's start at the beginning: conception.

As most everyone knows, all humans have two sex chromosomes. For women it's XX (an X from each parent), and for men it's XY (an X from mother and a Y from father). The father's contribution looks like a Y because it is literally missing one 'arm' of what would otherwise be an X-shaped chromosome. Who knows where or how the one arm of the Y chromosome got lost—it's probably buried somewhere out in the garage—but the missing fragment leaves the Y coming up short. Plenty short. The female X chromosome has 1,090 genes; the male Y chromosome has 80, and many of those are fairly routine housekeeping genes with the remaining few having to do with testicular and male development. To add insult to insufficiency, genes on the Y chromosome have twice the mutation frequency of those on the X chromosome, thank you very much.

What the bumbling, fumbling male sex chromosome does have that it can brag about is the SRY gene. It's the gene that encodes for a protein that instructs the sex area of the embryo to "go nuts," literally. In other words, Mother Nature made being female the default browser for fetal development. The cells are saying, "Unless we hear otherwise, we're painting the womb pink."

Should the SRY gene go trumpeting through the developing embryo, testosterone levels will peak in the second trimester at a level that parallels peak pubertal levels (fortunately, the confines of the uterus prevent the young male fetus from pulling some of the stunts he might well attempt as a testosterone-laden adolescent). Testosterone levels fall back to undetectable at birth, reach a smaller crest in the first few months of life, and then dive back to undetectable until puberty, at which point they peak again.

Most testosterone comes from—you guessed it—the testicles. The testes actually secrete three different male hormones, collectively known as androgens: testosterone, dihydrotestosterone, and androstenedione. From their perch atop the kidneys, the adrenal glands produce androgens in both men and women, but the amount is so small (less than 5 percent of adult male androgens) that even in women, the only masculinizing effect they have is to produce pubic and axillary (aka armpit) hair.

Once released into the bloodstream by the testicles, testosterone has an hour or two to either be absorbed into tissues and do something, or be deactivated and thrown into the recycling bin.

Like other hormones, testosterone is escorted around the body by certain proteins: 97 percent of testosterone is either loosely bound to the protein albumin, or more strongly bound to another protein called "sex hormone binding globulin." The forces that trigger the release of testosterone from its chaperone and into active duty are not well understood, and that complicates our understanding of what a "normal" testosterone level should be. It is clear that as men age, the amount of sex hormone binding globulin increases, thereby locking up more testosterone, perhaps to save us from ourselves.

Males carry about 20 percent of the amount of estrogen that a non-pregnant female does. Some is produced by the testicles, where the estrogen is thought to be important in sperm production. ("Where is your tail?" "What do you mean 'It was just here by the back door?'" "I don't care where you left it, or who had it last—you're not going out without your tail!")

The largest fraction of a man's estrogen levels, perhaps 80 percent, comes from conversion of testosterone to estrogen in other body tissues, particularly in the liver and in fat cells.

Men need estrogen for all kinds of reasons, but it's especially important in bone health. Case in point: a male friend of mine who was physically robust and active had a proclivity for breaking bones after only minor trauma. It turned out that he had low estrogen levels, owing to a lack of the aromatase enzyme that converts testosterone into estrogen.

Hormones Aren't the Half of It

So this is not an exclusive club: both men and women have estrogen and testosterone, albeit in different proportions. The testes make

7,000 ug of testosterone each day, but just 0.25 percent of that (or 17.5 ug) is converted to estrogen. The ovaries make just 300 ug of testosterone daily, but convert about half of that (or 150 ug) to estrogen.

Although it's easy to measure the blood levels of these flagship hormones, the story of how they impact a body is considerably more complicated.

What really matters is what happens when these hormones get inside individual cells and tissues. In that way, the role of hormones in gender archetypes has been oversimplified, as if light entering the eye were the only requisite for seeing. That light has to stimulate the cells of the retina, which convert the light into a neurological signal that can be sent to the brain to be interpreted and "seen."

Similarly, hormones are just the first signal in a cascade of events. They have to get inside a cell, either by passively diffusing across the cell wall or by binding to a receptor that will shuttle it—or its message—across the wall and into the cell. And when it does get inside the cell, the hormone has to activate the genes that will create proteins that will do its intended work. Complicating matters further, individual cells contain proteins—coactivators and corepressors—that can ramp up or tone down expression of the hormone.

"Nuanced" doesn't fully describe it. "Messy" might. What the messiness points out is that our individual genetic profile defines our individual sexuality more than our hormone levels do.

As Dr. Daniel Federman wrote in the *New England Journal of Medicine* in 2006, "Thus, each tissue can construct its own androgenic or estrogenic identity with developmental and potentially behavioral consequences that could not be predicted on the basis of circulating hormone levels."

Testosterone, the Extreme Makeover Edition
So what does testosterone do, physically, to a man?

It makes men hairy—on the face and the chest, with heavier hair on the arms and legs, and also the line of hair that trails down from the belly button to the pubic bone. This line of hair performs a critical homing beacon function when men need to locate their penis in the dark, or in a drunken stupor, or in a darkened drunken stupor. Or after a cold swim when everything has nearly disappeared courtesy of the cremasteric reflex.

No surprise, testosterone promotes the manufacture of male organs. The penis, scrotum, and testes enlarge about eight times under the rising testosterone levels of puberty. It deepens the male voice, and gives men thicker skin with more sebum—that is, more active oil glands, perhaps so that competing males can smell each other when they're approaching (acceding to the philosophy, "There's no such thing as bad PR").

Testosterone gives men more muscle. On average, men have about 50 percent more muscle mass than women, with beefier tendons and ligaments. And yes, thicker skulls, literally.

Sex on the Brain

And what does testosterone do to the male brain?

The idea that men think with their testicles is a complete and utter phallacy, as are those cartoon diagrams of the male brain, the ones that show a monstrously large portion of the brain being dedicated to "SEX, SPORTS, FOOD," with smaller peripheral portions beig cordoned off for "Spatial skills," "Toys and Tools," "Selective hearing," "Math," and "Building things." Areas dedicated to cooking and listening skills appear as tiny specks.

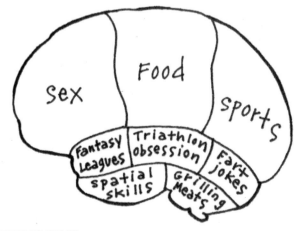

A word of caution here: this kind of catchy social media graphic is very misleading and does a great disservice to the study of male cognitive function, mainly because on a *real male brain* you wouldn't see any of these labels. Otherwise, it is probably accurate.

There's no doubt that male and female brains are different, and the difference starts right away, inside the uterus. Some of the variation is anatomical, and visible enough to detect on MRI scans in the first month of a newborn. We know that men are more likely to develop autism, Tourette's syndrome, and early onset schizophrenia, whereas women are more likely to develop depression, anxiety, and eating disorders. You may have heard that women's superior linguisitic skills reflect more robust development of the left-brain language centers, whereas men's advantage in spatial skills is consistent with more robust development of right-brain visual-spatial areas. Although that fits a certain narrative—women talk, men throw balls—the idea is still controversial.

Oddly enough, the joke that men think with their gonads parallels an old and fading theory of sexual brain development. If it carries the SRY gene, fetal gonadal tissue will transform itself into a testicle. Done. If it carries the SRY gene, fetal brain tissue will be wired up as a male brain. Done.

But surprise, the brain is far more complicated than a testicle, and epigenetics is one of the reasons why. Epigenetics looks at how different life experiences as well as dietary and chemical exposures can turn genes on and off, sometimes permanently. We think of genes as the definitive blueprint of our cells—a canon of edicts to be followed. But in fact, they are being interpreted, read, and edited by a very complex system of genetic enzymes and controls, some of which are influenced by the here-and-now. Why don't identical twins, with their identical DNA, become identical people? Epigenetics. Different experiences and different exposures made them different people.

As a disturbing and more speculative example of the role of epigenetics, I have a friend who spent part of his childhood in Connecticut, where he was exposed to excessively high levels of Yankees baseball fandom. Just a few years of insidious innoculation, and BOOM!, his sense of parity and let's-share-the-talent-to-make-the-game-more-interesting gene was turned completely off. Sinister but true.

Given how actively our brains interact with our environment, "the old noodle" has become an important focus for epigenetic research. Perhaps one day neuroscientists will be able to dissect out the startlingly complex influence that sex hormones and epigenetics have on brain and gender development. It's certainly more complicated than skirts for little girls, and pants for little boys. In the meantime, their work will likely continue to remind us that the pink brain and blue brain are vastly more similar than they are different.

Of course there are conditions where that is not always apparent. Tragically, the cause of the pervasive and crippling disease, Male Refrigerator Blindness ("Where is it?! ... it's not in here!") remains elusive.

GREAT SEXPECTATIONS

Clapping on, Clapping off: Erectile Dysfunction and the Rise of the Pecker Power Industry

During high school, I worked evenings in the dining area of an upscale retirement center. There were about 15 of us on each shift, and the working conditions were typically hot and steamy—in part due to the automatic dishwasher and the food warmers on the food line, but mostly because we were 16 and 17 and our sexual thermostats were all set on "high and horny."

We did our best to serve the elderly patrons in between all the flirting and teasing with our teenage co-workers, which was a full-time job itself. Despite all the hormones in the air, or maybe because of them, it never occurred to us to wonder how many of those retirees would be going upstairs after their meal and having sex. Never. Not once.

Should it matter to any of us how often other people are having sex? All that *should* matter is whether you and your partner feel satisfied with your sex life. Nevertheless, we're all a little curious about how the other half lives, because in the end, we'd all secretly like to feel that we are at least somewhere in the normal neighborhood, waiting for a bus on the corner of Typical and Average.

In 2005 to 2006, the National Social Life, Health, and Aging Project (NSHAP)

MAN OVERBOARD!

"Doing it" right: how often is often enough? You decide. Not sure how big a problem you have? Take the Sexual Health Inventory for Men quiz. Getting an erection is physiologically complicated. The brain is a sex organ. Pecker Power drugs do work. Side effects reasonable.

interviewed about 3,000 people, ages 57 to 85, about their sexual activity. Here are the results:

Prevalence of Sexual Behavior in Older Men and Women

	Sex at least once per year	Sex at least twice per month
Ages 57–64	84% men 62% women	55% men 41% women
Ages 65–74	67% men 40% women	44% men 26% women
Ages 75–85	39% men 17% women	21% men 9% women

Do those numbers sound right to you? Never mind the singular difficulty of imagining your parents, you know, *doing it*, even if doing it is what they needed to do to create you—you, who ended up *doing it* too. But the grandparents clapping on, clapping off up there in their senior living apartment? That's even harder.

Who knows what goes on behind closed doors, or in sex surveys, but do those numbers seem plausible to you? Perhaps this will help. The researchers defined sexual activity as "any mutually voluntary activity with another person that involves sexual contact, whether or not intercourse or orgasm occurs." So their definition of clapping on-and-off included everything from a rousing standing ovation to a quiet and respectful golf clap.

Many of the conclusions from the NSHAP study were not surprising. More health problems meant less sex; more men were sexually active in part because there were more aging widows than aging widowers; older age meant less sex and more problematic sex—erectile dysfunction, vaginal dryness, firing too early or not at all, painful sex.

In keeping with the stereotypical idea that women are passionate about passion (i.e., sex as the climax of a relationship), and men are passionate about sex (i.e., sex as a sport), 40 percent to 50 percent of older women in the study said they lacked interest in sex and 25 percent said they didn't find it pleasurable.

In contrast, about 28 percent of men said they lacked interest in sex, but only 4 percent to 7 percent said they didn't find it pleasurable, which is an odd juxtaposition—a significant number of men lacked interest, even though they found it pleasurable. Perhaps performance anxiety had something to do with the discrepancy: 25 percent to 30 percent of men admitted to such, more than double what women reported.

Hoisting the Mainsail

With no disrespect to the problem of vaginal dryness, erectile dysfunction is a little more complicated, as the mechanics of "hoisting the mainsail" are physiologically more complex than making sure the deck is slick.

The penis is made up of a spongy, cavernous collection of smooth muscle cells. At rest, these muscle cells sit in a contracted, clamped down state, but when stimulated by the parasympathetic nervous system, nitric oxide (not *nitrous* oxide, the active ingredient in "laughing gas") is released from the cells lining these small caverns. This causes the smooth muscles to relax, allowing blood to begin flowing into the caverns—the holes in the sponge so to speak.

As these areas expand, they pinch off the veins that normally drain the blood from this area. Blood flowing in but finding no way out causes the penis to enlarge and harden. Think of it as a hydraulic jack: hydraulic fluid being pumped in without a way out causes the pressure to rise.

There's a lot that can go wrong here. One can debate the merits of the claim that men think with their penises, but when it comes to this pinnacle of penile prowess—an erection—it really does all start in the brain.

There's an area deep in the brain, the locus ceruleus, that serves as the center for testosterone-dependent sexual arousal. As men age, there is less testosterone to stimulate this neurologic sexual command center, which also becomes less responsive over time. What was once a top-notch, elite Marine force eventually becomes a pudgy, out-of-shape group of Civil War reenactors. We don't think of the brain as a sex organ, but it is: it dictates who and how and when we find someone sexy, and it can also put the kibosh on the entire thing, for example, via depression, alcohol intoxication, or performance anxiety.

Nerve damage, often from diabetes, diminishes the triggering mechanism for an erection. And the same factors that cause atherosclerosis (diabetes, smoking, hypertension) can damage both the small arteries of the penis and the smooth muscle cells that trigger blood pooling and expansion to occur.

Do I Have ED, or Am I Just a Normal, Aging Silverback Male?

If you're on the fence about whether or not you have erectile dysfunction, why not take the International Index of Erectile Function quiz, or its more easily administered version with the whitewashed title, Sexual Health Inventory for Men (SHIM)? Because love is the international language in which erectile dysfunction is a form of bad grammar, SHIM has been translated into 30 languages.

The quiz involves only six questions, and the first asks men to rate their confidence in getting and keeping an erection. The other five boil down to something like, "How often can you create enough tensile strength, and maintain it long enough, to satisfy you and your partner?" A score of less than 22 (out of 30) suggests erectile dysfunction, and the lower the number, the worse it is. The SHIM I looked at recommended, "Discuss your answers with your doctor today," but really, one could probably just settle for the next available appointment.

The Rise of the Pecker Power Industry

Hallmark Pecker Power drugs like Viagra and Cialis and truck stop favorites like "Crankshaft" all contain phosphodiesterase type 5 inhibitors. The name references the enzyme they inhibit, thereby enhancing the way that the smooth muscle cells in the penis react to pro-arousal forces.

This ability to make smooth muscle cells relax is what led to the discovery of this class of erectile dysfunction drugs. Blood vessel walls are also made of smooth muscle, and so drugs that cause smooth muscle to loosen up will also cause blood vessels to dilate and enlarge—thereby lowering blood pressure. In the late 1980s and early 1990s, researchers at Pfizer were trying to develop a drug to treat angina (heart pain caused by poor blood flow) when they found that volunteers "complained" of increasing erections as a side effect. The rest is history—and the drug known first as UK-92480 (which sounds like something from the Soviet space program) became the blockbuster Viagra.

Erectile dysfunction screening tools like the SHIM might be useful for epidemiological and public health research, but I am not sure they make much difference to patients. Whatever the score, an unhappy man ends up in the doctor's office. Assuming that the initial workup doesn't show a reversible cause of ED, phosphodiesterase 5 inhibitors like Viagra (sildenafil) are widely prescribed on a trial basis, and if they seem to help, then the trial gets "extended."

> "They've done studies, you know.
> Sixty percent of the time,
> it works every time."
> —*Paul Rudd as Brian Fantana, Anchorman*

Who knows exactly what's in Fantana's Sex Panther cologne (other than "bits of real panther, so you know it's good"), but it brings us back to the idea that the brain is a sex organ. Because confidence means something.

A review of 14 trials in which patients were randomized to either sildenafil or placebo showed that although 78 percent of Viagra takers reported improvement in their erections, so did 25 percent of men who were taking the placebo (the placebo effect of *any* drug is a story in itself).

Another study took 123 men and divided them into three unblinded groups—i.e. they were told what they were getting. One group would get an ED drug, one would take either an ED drug or a pla-

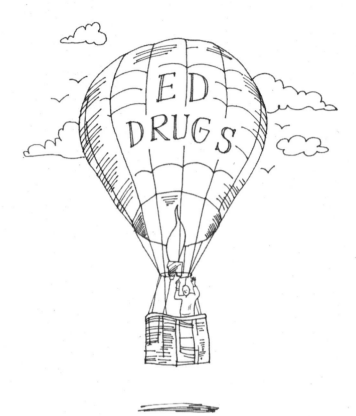

cebo, and one would receive a placebo. That's what the participants
were *told*, but what all three groups got was a placebo capsule full of
starch. (Is that even fair? I don't know.) In any case, after three months
of romance and starch, all three groups showed more than 30 percent
improvement in erectile function scores.

The point here? Pecker Power drugs do work, but they augment
a mechanical and physiological part of a complex process that has
strong and critical neurological and emotional inputs. They don't improve sensory nerve function and they don't work *directly* on the brain.
They're not aphrodisiacs, per se, but they can increase sexual drive by
decreasing performance anxiety with a confidence that affirms.

All of which leads a doctor colleague of mine to wryly conclude,
"They only work on the guys who don't need them."

No Drug Is Perfect: The Side Effects of Taking Big Rig

Back when ED drugs were new and their commercials ruled the airways, anyone with a television could list the side effects of these drugs from memory.

The most common side effects from ED drugs, starting with the most common, are headache, flushing, upset stomach, nasal congestion, vision problems (including a blue tinting), diarrhea, dizziness, and rash. Ironically, the list is eerily similar to the things you were warned in junior high would happen if you masturbated too much—minus the hair growth on the palms.

But it's the rare and serious side effects that grab our attention: the erection lasting more than four hours (Call the doctor? Call the neighbors!), a sudden loss of vision in one or both eyes, or a sudden loss of hearing.

The concerns about hearing and vision loss are self-explanatory: That ain't right. But what about the nonstop erection—termed "priapism" in medical speak? Hasn't a perpetual erection been the mythical stud goal since the beginning of time?

The intense pain of an overly sustained erection is a clue that this goal was a false one. Most episodes of priapism are painful, and the pain is not only due to the swelling but also because the penis is not getting enough oxygen. The high venous pressure inside the penis keeps new arterial blood from entering, and so oxygen levels dip. If the pressure and venous congestion goes on long enough, tissue damage— cell death—can occur. Scarring and—guess what? ED—are long-term complications.

Not to fear: priapism is a rare event. Roughly 5-8 of every 100,000 male visits to the emergency department are for a priapistic event, and some of those cases are from diseases or medications that have nothing to do with ED. More than 85 percent of those men were treated— almost certainly with a bag of ice to the crotch, and probably a few injections of reversal medications into the penis—and then released. A small number needed to be admitted to the hospital for more treatment, in some cases a surgical decompression to release the pressure. Imagine that. Or maybe don't.

Although the idea of a four-hour erection certainly sticks in the public imagination, perhaps the biggest issue with the Pecker Power medications is that they can cause a drop in blood pressure. This dip is usually quite modest and of no consequence in an otherwise healthy individual. But many men with ED have significant atherosclerotic disease—that's how they developed ED in the first place. And to cloud this issue further, some heart medications—nitrates and alpha-blockers in particular—can exacerbate this drop in blood pressure.

The idea of newly empowered ED sufferers passing out or dropping dead from a heart attack while in the middle of intercourse was not good for early sales of drugs like "The Shortshank Redemption." But since then, numerous studies have found that ED drugs do not increase the risk of dying from a heart attack, even if the user has heart disease. Nitrates (aka nitroglycerin), the little dissolvable pills that can be slipped under the tongue to chase away chest pain, are still kind of a no-no right around the time you're using ED drugs, as are blood pressure–lowering alpha-blockers.

Sex can still break your heart—the act itself does seem to carry a transient increase in heart attack risk—but if you need a couple of tablets of Crankshaft in the old belly before turning the lights down low, the odds are in your favor that everything will turn out just fine. Alternatively, you can try a starch capsule.

BALD IS BEAUTIFUL, BUT IS IT UNHEALTHY?

Is Hair Loss a Disease or a "Condition"? And What to Do—or Not to Do—about It?

There are two uniquely male experiences: getting hit in the testicles so hard that you feel like you're never going to inhale again, and going bald. Granted, on rare occasions women go bald, and the rarity of it makes the angst 10 times higher. But even a woman with thinning hair will never have the experience of falling off her bike and getting racked in the ovaries.

When it comes to balding, I've clearly got some skin in the game. I was in my early 20s when I first felt a raindrop hit the top of my head in an unusually direct fashion. I remember the moment vividly. The raindrop didn't pinball down a number of hair follicles and then slowly seeeeeeep onto my scalp. It hurtled straight through my thinning hair and crash-landed on my scalp with the sound of someone thumping a melon in the produce aisle. It was a new sensation, but one I would get used to.

Since this is not a book about societal norms, I'll leave out any discussion about whether the truck stop T-shirt "Bald Is Beautiful" is correct, other than to say that Michael Jordan did more to pump up the

MAN OVERBOARD!

Bald may or may not be beautiful, but it isn't a disease. Susceptible hair follicles are genetically programmed to shrink away when exposed to androgens. Lotions and pills work best for mild to moderate thinning; if you stop, all gains are lost. Transplantation is safe but $pendy. Comb-over illegal in 37 states and the District of Columbia.

sagging egos of the National Balding Association than he did to revitalize the National Basketball Association. Although Jordan won six NBA championships, history will one day remember him for a much more significant feat: popularizing the clean-shaved head, thereby vanquishing the contemptible and hideous comb-over—the scalp scourge that has plagued mankind since the invention of Brylcreem. Bless you, Michael Jordan.

One thing's for sure: it is much easier to *be* bald than it is to *go* bald. The process is a distressing, painfully slow cosmetic change that undeniably ages you. And the thinning period is when a lot of people feel like they want to make some comment about your hairline, like it's a sudoku puzzle and they're the first one to figure it out. People don't say, "Hey, I see you're getting a little pudgy around the neck!" or, "You know, I'm noticing that your butt is struggling against the tyranny of your pants," but they'll comment on your balding with a certain irritating righteousness—as if to spare you some embarrassment, as if they were pointing out a booger hanging off your nose that you hadn't noticed. You'd like to shave their heads clean and plunk their noggins like melons until they come to their senses.

Hakuna Ma-Hair-Follicle

There is a cycle of life for every hair, and here it is: all of us start out with roughly 100,000 terminal hair follicles on our scalps. These are different from the follicles that build the lighter, shorter hair found on the rest of our body. At any given time, about 90 percent to 95 percent of these terminal hair follicles are in a growth phase that lasts anywhere from two to six years (longer growth time means longer hair). This is followed by a two-to-three-week involution stage, when the base of the follicle—the manufacturing end of things—goes into physiologic foreclosure. A "resting phase" follows, in which no additional hair length is manufactured. After two to three months, the hair falls out and the follicle starts all over again. Every day, about 100 hairs die off and 100 sprout up.

The forces that control this hairy cycle are "complex," a word doctors and researchers use when they don't understand what's going on.

It just sounds better, more scientific. For example, "My feelings for you are complex" certainly sounds better than "I have no idea what our relationship means to me." See?

It's clear that androgens, like testosterone, send strong messages to the hair follicles. When puberty comes awkwardly calling, androgens stimulate follicles in the beard, chest, legs and arms to put out stockier, thicker hair; and conversely, it causes follicles in the temples to put out smaller-caliber, finer hair (not to split hairs, but this isn't hair loss in terms of numbers of hairs, but rather in terms of volume of hair).

In male pattern hair loss ("androgenetic alopecia" in medicalese), susceptible hair follicles in certain areas of the scalp cower under the biochemical influence of testosterone and its more active metabolite dihydrotestosterone. Over time, these follicles produce a flimsier and flimsier product—thinner in diameter and shorter in length, so that hair that used to stand tall and thick like an oak tree now looks like orchard grass. If you're bald, these are the pesky remnant little hairs that can evade even the sharpest clippers, only to spring up antenna-like later on.

The genetic basis of balding is also "complex." But it is definitely inherited—we can say that with certainty. Inherited through your genes. Via your parents. In a way that is "complex," and that involves a number of genes, and not just one Big Bald Gene. Whatever the Androgenetic Alopecia Gene Pack is, it must have something to do with how hair follicles respond to dihydrotestosterone (DHT)—a potent metabolite of testosterone that is responsible for many of the masculinizing effects of testosterone. That's because blocking the conversion of testosterone to DHT stops the balding process, and because balding men have normal blood levels of testosterone and other male hormones (there goes the Hyper-virile Theory of Balding).

Do I Have a Disease?

I strongly adhere to the principle that bald is beautiful—if beauty is in the eye of the beholder, and the beholder thinks a clean, uncluttered scalp is beautiful.

But vendors of balding remedies seem to favor the diseased view, peppering the airwaves with language that instructs me that I am, for example, "suffering from a progressive condition called male pattern hair loss" (as opposed to suffering from a progressive condition called multiple sclerosis, or Alzheimer's, or what have you). They tell me that losing my hair is "not normal," but reassure me, "You're not alone," because millions of other men have this not-normal condition.

An ad from a local sportscaster here in the Twin Cities proclaimed, "More hair, more life!" which finally forced me to admit that what I'm really dealing with is a *life deficit*. All of these ads imply that this isn't about my personal appearance: I have a disease and I need to treat it.

Is being bald truly a health concern? In 2013, researchers from Tokyo University tried to clarify the strength of a previously recognized association (which isn't the same as causation) between male pattern baldness and heart disease. Yes, hair loss increases one's risk of getting skin cancer of the dome, but does it really increase the chance that you'll have a heart attack?

They pored through six studies that together included nearly 37,000 participants.

Let's say it again—association is no proof of causation—so don't lunge for the Rogaine, but for men of all ages, severe balding seemed to increase the risk of developing heart disease by 32 percent. The risk was higher—44 percent—for men who developed severe baldness before their mid- to late 50s.

Several of the studies the researchers reviewed used the Hamilton-Norwood scale of balding, which, with all due respect to Hamilton and Norwood, I had never heard of before. It was interesting to find that balding can be more objectively categorized than the informal scale I've been using:

The Dr. Craig Bowron Scale of Balding
Stage 1: Thinning
Stage 2: Getting breezy
Stage 3: Deep denial but I admire the effort
Stage 4: Comfortably bald (to the tune of
Pink Floyd's classic "Comfortably Numb")

Using the more official Hamilton-Norwood scale, they found that hair loss at the vertex—the part of the skull where a beanie or yarmulke would be placed—carried the strongest association with heart disease. The more severe the vertex hair loss, the higher the risk: 18 percent for mild, 36 percent for moderate, and 48 percent for severe. On the other hand, a receding hairline held no statistically significant association.

Why the association? Are our solar sex panels somehow absorbing mysterious atherosclerosis-causing radiation from the sun? The authors of the study admitted that the mechanism for any connection between heart disease and balding remains unclear.

Here's how I see it: anyone who has risk factors for heart disease (smoking, high cholesterol, diabetes, hypertension) should address them, because there is plenty of evidence that controlling your blood pressure, for example, can lower your risk of having a heart attack. But there's no evidence that treating your hair loss can do the same (although there is some evidence that a comb-over can increase your heart disease risk, simply by irritating God).

Lotions and Potions

If your scalp is receding like a Greenland glacier and you're serious about fighting it, minoxidil lotion and finasteride pills are the mainstay of medical therapy.

Minoxidil (Rogaine) was one of the first to be available. Although it was initially used to treat high blood pressure, minoxidil segued into a much more successful second career as a friend to the hair impaired after it was found to have hair regeneration as a side effect.

It works. Hair follicles produce thicker and longer hair, and "hair weights" (the amount of hair in a specified area of the scalp) increase by an average of around 30 percent. It's not clear precisely how minoxidil actually promotes hair growth—there are plenty of other medications that dilate blood vessels like minoxidil does, but they don't stimulate hair growth.

Finasteride (Propecia) blocks the conversion of testosterone into the more active dihydrotestosterone (DHT), the hormone that causes hair follicles to shrink. Finasteride causes levels of DHT in the scalp and the blood to drop by as much as 60 percent. Fortunately, the small number of patients who note decreased libido and erectile dysfunction at the initiation of therapy find that these side effects dissipate quickly. Finasteride doesn't seem to work as well in men in their sixties, probably because their levels of the DHT enzyme are already falling. For older men in particular, it works best when there are still some miniaturized hairs left to be revived.

For both minoxidil and finasteride, patience is a virtue: you're growing hair, not a Chia pet. With minoxidil, it can take two to three months to see appreciable results, and one might even see some increased hair shedding before that. Don't panic: it's temporary. With finasteride, it can take 6 to 12 months to see significant improvement in turf coverage.

It's important to have realistic expectations: you'll never get back to the mane you had sophomore year in high school, and the farther along you are in the balding process, the less effective these medications will be. It's as if the follicles are sleeping too deeply to be awakened. And like the disclaimer you often hear, individual results may vary: most users have hair growth, but for some, the drugs just maintain what you already have.

Perhaps the biggest drawback to these hair loss drugs is that when you stop using them, your pilgrim's progress falls out and you're back to where you would have been in a matter of months.

If you want to go for the Trifecta of Hair Growth, you'll need to purchase a laser hat. It sounds like something out of the military—"On evening patrols, be sure to have your night-vision goggles and your laser hat"—but the technology uses lower-level lasers to penetrate the scalp and reactivate hair follicles. You can buy it as a hat, helmet, cap, comb, and headband. Ads for laser therapy devices sometimes proclaim their product to be "FDA Approved"—that is, approved by the US Food and Drug Administration—or "FDA Cleared," but that applies to safety and not to whether they are effective. It seems likely that they do work, and that they work best for those with mild to moderate hair loss. However, the International Society of Hair Restoration Surgery has taken no official stand on laser therapy, citing lack of large well-designed, double-blind studies. One small study stands out in my mind, not because of its results, which showed laser therapy to be effective, but because it was published in the *Indian Journal of Dermatology, Venereology, and Leprology*—an entirely different trifecta.

One last option: scalp micropigmentation (SMP). It uses an electric tattoo device to add pigment into areas of hair loss.

Hair Transplantation (Pronounced "Hair Tran$plantation")

The impermanent effect of hair loss medications is one thing that makes the permanency of hair transplantation so enticing. The name is an accurate description of the procedure: hair follicles that are not sensitive to dihydrotestosterone—the ones on the side of the head— are transplanted (or "grafted") to the areas of the scalp where the DHT-sensitive follicles are still living out their flimsy existence.

There are two primary methods for hair transplantation: follicular unit extraction (FUE) and follicular unit transplantation (FUT). The FUE process is a bit like a greenskeeper changing the hole location on a green: a tiny plug of hair (0.8 to 0.1 mm in diameter and containing one to four hair follicles) is extracted 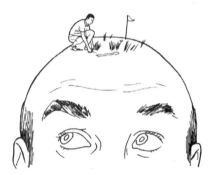 from hairy scalp and replanted in a bald area. The donor site hole heals closed. FUT is sometimes referred to as follicular unit "strip" surgery, because a strip of donor hair is removed from the back of the scalp. The incision is sutured closed, and the strip of hair is divided into graft units containing 1-4 hairs. FUE is newer, has a quicker recovery time, and does not leave a linear scar, but FUT offers the densest coverage.

Typically a patient can get good coverage with two to four transplantation sessions, but of course that depends on how much "green" needs to be covered. Speaking of green, the procedure is quite spendy— typically in the $8K to 12K range *per session*. Some hair tran$plantation surgeons go as high as $20K per session, but I am told you can get it for

$2K in Turkey (which includes a free off-market laser cap and a year's subscription to the *Indian Journal of Dermatology, Venereology, and Leprology*).

If you're horrified by that price tag, consider the barbaric procedures that hair tran$plantation has replaced. How about "scalp reduction surgery"? I am not making this up. A plastic surgeon, or any surgeon in Tijuana, would surgically remove bare scalp at the back of the head and then sew the area closed by pulling in adjacent hair-bearing scalp. The technique didn't work on the frontal hairline because the surgeon couldn't exactly pull your face up to cover the hole, unless you've got the shrub-like eyebrows of Eugene Levy. That might work.

The other aggressive option was "flap surgery," which is the surgical form of the dreaded comb-over. Rather than combing freakishly long strands of hair from one side of the head over the bald spot and then gluing them down with hair tonic or epoxy, flap surgery involves loosening up a section of hair-bearing scalp (a "flap") from the side of the head and then rotating it forward and sewing it in place. Assuming it's sewn down tight and heals well, a surgical flap is more resistant to wind shear and derision than the traditional comb-over.

Since male pattern hair loss is considered a cosmetic—not medical—issue, surgical options are typically an out-of-pocket expense. This can be offset by putting your collection of balding-themed T-shirts, hats, and coffee mugs up for sale on eBay: "Wish You Were Hair," "Who Needs Hair with a Body Like This?" "Male Pattern Awesomeness," "Struggling Hair Farmer," or the "It's Not a Bald Spot; It's a Solar Panel for a Sex Machine" sweatshirt that she'll never let you wear.

Or you could purchase *Man Overboard!*'s more scientifically minded sloganwear: "I've Got a Polyglycine-Encoding GGN Repeat in Exon 1 of My Androgen-Receptor Gene. What's Your Excuse?"

Like many societal norms, the desirability or disability of being bald is really a matter of perspective, and I think we're coming around on this one. I see progress. Comb-overs and toupees seem to be fading into the past, and bald men have come to understand that fully coiffed men deserve neither our sympathy nor derision: it's genetic—they were born that way.

For men, it's like the brain's like, "Every month I got to grow hair on this guy's head, Every month I got to grow hair on this guy's head"... and then one month the brain's like, "Every month I got to grow hair everywhere *but* this guy's head."

—*Jim Gaffigan on*
The Late Show with Stephen Colbert

5 LOW BACK PAIN

Do You Do the Lumbago? If You Haven't, You Probably Will

The human spine has a lot in common with human parents: it has to be supportive and firm, yet somehow remain flexible. It has to be protective of the delicate little neurons that make up the spinal cord, but it also has to allow them to venture out into the world, or how can they do their own thing? And how many times, dear parents, has the spinal cord come back to express gratitude to the bony spine? Nay, not once. Or rarely.

But back to the spine, which is made up of seven cervical vertebrae in the neck, twelve thoracic vertebrae in the chest, and five lumbar vertebrae in what's typically referred to as the "low back" region.

Looking down on a vertebra, it has the appearance of an oval rock with a squat Japanese pagoda perched on top of it. The pagoda has two short sidewalls, and a roof line that slopes to a spiny peak—which is what you feel when you run your fingers down the spine. Inside the pagoda lies the sacred text—the spinal cord—which is connected to (more accurately, a continuation of) the Mighty Melon, the human brain.

Every vertebra has this basic structure,

MAN OVERBOARD!

Behold the spine, bearer of weight, strong but flexible. Discs herniate and pinch nerves—wham! Joints become arthritic, swollen, and inflamed and then pinch nerves—ouch! Most episodes of low back pain will resolve on their own. Without evidence of infection, tumor, serious weakness, or loss of contact with Phil Nether, a CT scan or MRI can wait. Treatments are aimed primarily at pain relief, reducing inflammation and swelling, and passing time while the body heals. Remain calm. Keep moving. Stay patient. In almost every case, surgery is NOT the first, or second, or third option.

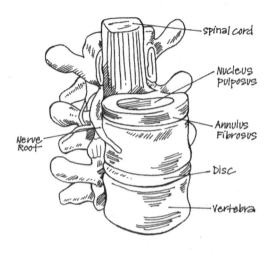

spinal cord

Nucleus
Pulposus

Annulus
Fibrosus

Nerve
Root

Disc

Vertebra

with variations based on the level of the spine it occupies. Lumbar vertebrae are bulkier because they are at the bottom of the spine and support the most weight; the cervical vertebrae in the neck are the lightest.

The oval-shaped base of each vertebra is what supports the weight of the spine, and the vertebrae are separated from one other by a cushiony disc that in some ways resembles a Hostess Ding Dong. Rather than a hurricane-proof, chocolate-flavored, paraffin outer shell, the disc has a gristly cartilaginous cover called the "annulus fibrosus"; replacing the creamy synthetic filling is a softer, squishier middle called the "nucleus pulposus."

Although there's something shabbily delectable about a Ding Dong metaphor, these spinal discs are closer to a gel seat for your bicycle—a tough outer shell protecting a gelatinous core that is designed to cush' the tush.

When some poor soul suffers a "slipped disc," it means that a split or tear in the tougher outer layer of the disc has allowed the softer center to bulge into the area inside the pagoda, where the sacred spinal cord is housed. A more accurate descriptor, rather than "slipped" or "bulging" (like waistlines, it's common for discs to bulge some as they age), is "herniated."

If this herniated disc pushes on one of the nerves as it exits the spine and heads down to the legs, it causes an excruciating, electric zinger-type pain that shoots into the buttocks and legs. This pain is called "sciatica" (pronounced sigh-AT-i-cuh) because it often involves the sciatic nerve—the longest nerve in the body, which innervates most of the muscles of the leg.

If the herniation in the dinged-up Ding Dong disc is so large that it compresses the spinal cord itself, then you've got bigger problems: all of the nerves from that disc level down can be compromised by the pressure, leading to weakness in both legs. It can also lead to loss of sensation and function in what doctors often call the "nether regions," (after British anatomist and explorer Dr. Phil Nethers, who first discovered them on an expedition to the Central Groin region in 1833).

The lamina of each vertebra is the roof of the spinal canal, which interlocks with the roof of the vertebrae above and below it. This means the spine contains a whopping 44 joints—about what you'd find in the tour bus of a Grateful Dead cover band. These so-called "facet joints" are similar to other joints in the body in that they are covered in cartilage and surrounded by a capsule that keeps a small amount of lubricating fluid in the joint. But facet joints don't allow anywhere near the range of motion seen with other joints; instead, they serve a basic hinge-like function. To provide additional strength, the individual vertebrae are lashed together by a variety of ligaments and muscles.

Do You Do the Lumbago?

Lumbago (lum-BAY-go) is one of the terms used to describe low back pain, but it sounds more like a Chilean folk dance—or a maneuver you'd learn about in an underwater birthing class.

Chances are, at some unfortunate point in your life, you will learn to do the lumbago: after skin problems and arthritis, low back pain is the third most common reason for a visit to the doctor's office. Maybe you'll be able to tough it out at home for a while, but if you finally end up going into the office, you'll be hoping that your doctor can figure out what's causing the pain and concoct a plan to make it go away or, at the very least, figure out how to turn off the pesky Chilean folk music you keep hearing in your head.

What, Exactly, Is the Problem?

Let's get this over with and be disappointed right now, while you're not in pain. It's simpler that way.

The spine is structurally so complex that it's often very difficult to tell *what exactly* is the source of a patient's low back pain—a torn and/or herniated disc, an injured muscle or ligament, an inflamed facet joint? The physical exam is often not very helpful, and blood testing is even less so.

Doctors can and do order CT or MRI scans to try to convey that we are scientifically and emotionally invested in your problem. But we also understand that by the time you get the scan and make a follow-up appointment, chances are you'll already be feeling better, and you will attribute this improvement to the kind and empathetic way in which we listened to your soul-weary lumbago story.

Early CT or MRI imaging of the low back is generally frowned upon in low back pain care guidelines because these "let's take a peek, just to be sure" tests rarely, if ever, change the initial treatment approach. Too often they raise more questions (and patients' anxiety levels) than they answer. That's because the aging human spine accrues all kinds of subtle and not-so-subtle signs of wear and tear. Most of these nicks and scrapes and lumps and bumps aren't causing any problems. Studies of MRI scans on people with no history of back pain commonly show arthritis, ligament damage, bulging-but-not-herniated discs, and pinched nerves—yet they have no pain. The big picture question isn't, "Does my back look showroom-new?" because in most cases it will certainly not. The question is: Is there anything on the MRI that clearly explains your signs and symptoms, and if so, is it something that requires immediate intervention? The answer is: Typically not, and you'll almost certainly get better on your own. In fact, you might even recover quicker without the MRI findings freaking you out.

What about a simple X-ray? Those are easy to do in the office, where they can be a good, low-cost screening tool. But because a plain X-ray sees only bones (and bony changes due to arthritis), it can't reveal much about the health of discs, ligaments, or pinched nerves.

Are there types of back pain that do require earlier imaging? Yes. Anyone with a history of recent trauma, or who has developed significant weakness in the legs or numbness in the Phil Nether regions, or who has a prior history of cancer (which rarely originates in the spine but sometimes starts elsewhere and then spreads to the spine), or whose presentation raises concern for a spinal infection (fever, HIV infection, or history of IV drug use) should get early imaging.

The incidence of these more serious things is pretty low—cancer and infection make up less than 1 percent of all the things that cause low back pain. But, no surprise: the risk of these more serious things goes up with age, so scanning earlier is more often indicated in older patients.

Now That We Don't Know What This Is, How Long Will It Take to Get Better?

Weren't you listening? I just told you what it is, *most likely*: if the pain is just in the low back, and not shooting down into the legs, then it's "mechanical low back pain." You can call it a "lumbar strain" or "lumbar sprain," but if you really want to impress your co-workers and friends, tell them you have "spondylosis." This is a more technical and empathy-producing term for the degenerative wear and tear of the back that comes with aging.

And it's almost certainly going to get better! About a third of people are substantially improved in one week, and two-thirds are substantially improved at seven weeks. Forty percent of the time the pain returns within six months, which might herald a more chronic low back pain condition. That doesn't mean the sufferer will become significantly disabled; it just portends a future with intermittent exacerbations. As with chronic conditions such as diabetes or high blood pressure, it might be a problem that one has to learn to live with and control.

If the problem is a slipped disc, with an Attack-o'-Sciatica, these also tend to improve, slowly, on their own. At about six weeks out, only about 10 percent of patients have persistent pain, and then surgery might be considered. Attack-o'-Sciatica accompanied by significant muscle weakness is a more ticklish issue and might require earlier surgery, which I will discuss a little later.

Acute Low Back Pain: Things to Do While Your Back Heals Itself

Let's start with what not to do: bed or couch rest. This approach went out with bloodletting for fevers and lobotomies for clinical depression. Inactivity makes everything worse. The muscles and ligaments in and around the injured area tighten up and add to the pain; the rest of the body goes to flab, the catnapping keeps you from sleeping well, and the brain develops what neurologists now call "Netflix Dementia." A couch-bound person with decent Internet access can become severely overentertained, a crippling condition that can sometimes require emergent detoxification with C-Span videos from the early '80s.

So you need to get up and get moving. Remember, motion is lotion and if you rest, you rust (available on T-shirt, hoodie, or cap in *Man Overboard!* swag section). Try to maintain your usual activities. You can do some light stretching, but don't go all Testostero and dial up aggressive boot-camp style calisthenics thinking you're gonna muscle your way out of this mess. It will only make the pain worse.

Then what? In 2017, the American College of Physicians reviewed all of the strongest clinical trials on therapies for low back pain to create a series of best-evidence clinical guidelines. Here's a list of things they thought were beneficial:

Acute Low Back Pain:

Nonsteroidal anti-inflammatory drugs (NSAIDs), skeletal muscle relaxants, heat wraps, massage, acupuncture, and spinal manipulation.

Chronic Low Back Pain:

Start with non-drug therapy options such as exercise, multidisciplinary rehab, acupuncture, mindfulness-based stress reduction, tai chi, yoga, motor control exercise, progressive relaxation, electromyography feedback, low-level laser therapy, operant therapy, cognitive behavioral therapy, or spinal manipulation. If those are ineffective, drug therapy options include NSAIDs, tramadol or duloxetine (an antidepressant).

Of note, most of these were deemed to be of small benefit, and none was better than "moderately beneficial." The smaller number of treatment options for those with acute (less than a month) or subacute (4 to 12 weeks) pain reflects the reality that most sufferers will recover relatively "quickly" anyway (easy for me to say). And it also explains why the list of treatment options for those with chronic pain is a whole lot longer.

Let's clarify a few items on the list:

Nonsteroidal Anti-Inflammatory Drugs (NSAIDs)

These are medications such as ibuprofen (aka Motrin, Advil), naproxen (aka Aleve, Naprosyn), and celecoxib (Celebrex) that work by providing analgesia (pain relief) and by decreasing the amount of inflammation around the area of the spine that your hapless doctor cannot or will not specifically identify (ask again to hear their "why-don't-I-need-an-MRI?" spiel). NSAIDs can be highly effective pain and inflammation relievers, but if used regularly, they can increase the risk of a heart attack or stroke, cause stomach ulcers, or interfere with kidney function. The risk of all of those things increases with higher doses, and with prolonged use. For patients with known cardiovascular disease, a short course of either naproxen or celecoxib is probably the safest option. For those without cardiovascular issues, the risk is so minimal that most doctors are comfortable prescribing any NSAID. Most patients with mildly weak kidneys will do fine with an occasional dosing; if you have significant kidney issues, check with your doctor first. NSAIDs can also increase the risk of bleeding. Usually the change is trivial, but for patients who are on other anticoagulants (aspirin, Plavix, or drugs like warfarin, Eliquis, or Xarelto) it can be enough to cause problems.

Acetaminophen Is in a "Class by Itself," So to Speak

Acetaminophen (Tylenol) is a common pain reliever, but it's not classified as an NSAID because it doesn't reduce inflammation. Perhaps that's why some consider it to be a less effective pain reliever than ibuprofen or naproxen. Even so, it's probably worth keeping acetaminophen on the "give this a whirl" list for low back pain, in part because it doesn't have any of the ulcer risks, kidney problems, or bleeding issues that NSAIDs do.

The major potential side effect of acetaminophen is liver injury, but that's very rare unless one has underlying liver problems or is consistently taking more than six to eight extra-strength tablets per day. (Extra-strength tablets are 500 mg, so 3,000 to 4000 mg per day is the safe ceiling.)

Steroidal Anti-Inflammatory Drugs

The mirror image to nonsteroidal anti-inflammatory drugs (NSAIDs) is steroidal anti-inflammatory drugs. You won't find them on the above list, but they are widely prescribed. These are not the kind of performance-enhancing steroids that will allow you to get a home run off a checked swing. These are the kind of steroids that reduce the inflammatory response to the initial injury. They can be taken as pills, or they can be injected into whatever area of the spine is causing trouble—a degenerating disc, an arthritic facet joint, or near (but not into!) an irritated and swollen nerve via an epidural steroid injection.

Skeletal Muscle Relaxants (SMR)

Tightening up muscles is nature's way of limiting the motions that are triggering pain. But if those muscles get too tight for too long, they can begin to spasm and increase the pain. Muscle relaxants (even physicians typically leave out the "skeletal" part) do exactly that—they relax tight muscles. But they also make people sleepy and you might miss something important on Netflix. Medications like Valium—known better as an old-timey anxiety reliever—can also be used to relax muscles. SMRs are really for short-term use. Ultrasound and massage therapy are probably better options for loosening up muscles and they have no side effects.

I Don't See "Chiropractors" on That List. Can They Help?

The answer is that as the main purveyors of "spinal manipulation" therapy, they are on the list, sort of; and yes, they can help.

According to the National Institutes of Health, every year about 10 percent of US adults seek out chiropractic care, where they are commonly treated with a technique called "spinal manipulation"—what many would call "an adjustment."

Spinal manipulation involves applying a controlled thrust—either by hand or with a device—to one or more joints of the spine.

In the ACP's guidelines for acute low back pain, spinal manipulation was one of only four interventions that had enough evidence to make the cut. The benefit was small, with 10 to 20 percent improvement in pain. In acute low back pain, chiropractors will often avoid or dial down their use of spinal manipulation in favor of massage and other techniques. Spinal manipulation is also recommended therapy for subacute and chronic low back pain.

Is spinal manipulation safe? Yes. The most common side effects—increased soreness, stiffness, or pain—are temporary, and the ACP found that the chance of spinal manipulation causing the underlying condition to worsen was exceedingly rare, less than one in a million.

A couple of notes:

- Doctors of Osteopathy (they have a DO behind their names) have the same medical training as M.D.s, but they have additional training in chiropractic techniques like spinal manipulation.
- Although the ACP reviewers cautioned that very few trials focused just on patients with sciatica (shooting nerve pain into the legs) or spinal stenosis, spinal manipulation seemed to work with or without sciatic symptoms.

What about Physical Therapists? They Aren't on the List Either.

Physical therapists are a common and critical resource for low back pain sufferers. Just like chiropractors, they don't appear on the list by name, but they do provide a number of the therapies (exercise, massage, electrical stimulation, rehab) noted on the list. Some are trained in spinal manipulation as well.

Since there is no one therapy regimen that works for everyone, a good physical therapist will customize a therapy plan for each patient (and alter it if needed).

When to See a Chiropractor or Physical Therapist

Probably sooner than later. There's good evidence that doing so gets people on the road to recovery sooner, while significantly reducing costs. For most patients with a flare of low back pain, a visit to a chiropractor or physical therapist will be far more useful than seeing a spine surgeon.

Opioids for Pain Relief: Welcome to the Jungle

Narcotics (opioids) are a highly addictive and dangerous quagmire.

In case you missed it, before the COVID-19 pandemic arrived in 2020, we were well into our second decade of an opioid overdose epidemic. It started with prescription narcotics such as OxyContin in the late '90s; the second wave came with a resurgence of heroin use around 2010; and a third wave, starting around 2015, was fueled by synthetic (manufactured in a lab) opioids such as fentanyl—the drug that ended the lives of Prince and Tom Petty, both of whom were taking it (apparently) for arthritic pain.

The fact that a popular opioid like fentanyl is available both by prescription and nefariously off the street makes it difficult to separate prescription-related overdoses from non-prescription deaths, but the Centers for Disease Control and Prevention (CDC) estimates that from 1999 to 2019, more than 247,000 Americans died from an overdose of prescription opioids.

Doctors—we who vowed to "do no harm"—were obviously complicit in this. Although a very small number of unscrupulous doctors saw the millions of Americans dealing with chronic pain as a business opportunity, the rest of us were swept up in a well-intentioned but misguided effort to make pain the "fifth vital sign." Blood pressure, pulse, temperature, breathing rate, *pain level*. Fueled by the pharmaceutical industry influence, it became vital that we keep our patients as comfortable as possible, whatever the consequences. So we prescribed narcotics for more people, at higher doses, for longer periods, and the results were disastrous. Fortunately, opioid prescribing rates have been declining since 2012, although according to the CDC, in 2017 more than 17% of Americans had at least one opioid prescription filled, averaging 3.4 prescriptions dispensed per patient. There is work to be done.

Obviously, an overdose death is the worst possible side effect of an opioid, but here are the most common ones:

- Nausea
- Constipation
- Drowsiness
- Confusion or delirium

Although we still encourage our hospitalized patients to "stay ahead of your pain," many find that they would rather deal with the pain than with the side effects of pain medications.

Choosing Opioids for Pain Is a Value Proposition: What Will I Get, and What Will It Cost Me?

We have to acknowledge that pain doesn't kill people, but pain pills can and do. That may sound crass, or just brutally honest, but when we are making choices between pain and pain treatment, we have to think clearly.

Brain Pain: Pain Is All in Our Heads, and Yet It Isn't

When I was suffering with a kidney stone, I could tell you *exactly* where my pain was coming from, and it wasn't anywhere near my head. I was not imagining my pain. And yet my brain was very much involved. A quote from pain specialist Dr. Howard Schubiner succinctly summarizes decades of pain research: "All pain is real, and all pain is generated by the brain."

The act of hearing is a good analogy to this brain pain theory. In the strictest sense, our ears hear nothing. They only convert the mechanical energy of different sound waves into a neurological impulse and then transmit that information to the brain. Then your brain decides what you're hearing—a crow in the distance, someone typing in the next room, the furnace turning on. The ear can't tell you what you're hearing. Only the brain can do that. The pain fibers scattered throughout our body collect injury and inflammation data and transmit that back to the brain, which interprets its source, severity, and implications.

Pain is a mix of the physical and the psychological. On rare occasions, people are born without pain receptors, and they feel no pain (to their detriment; pain sensations help us avoid injuries). But it's the brain that puts our pain in context, gives it meaning, and decides what emotional response should be attached to it. All of that is influenced by our own personal psychological stew—our past experiences with pain, our current stressors, our support network of family and friends, how we've learned to cope with adversity. When little children fall at the playground, they often look to their parent with a certain "How should I feel?" face, as if they are trying to decide whether to cry or not. Some parents sweep in and call for a medevac chopper, others ignore or dismiss ("Aw, you're fine!"), and some help the child debrief ("What happened? Where does it hurt? Let me see").

In the end, pain is very personal and very subjective. It isn't *all* in our heads, but a lot of it is. Without a doubt, our perception of pain is greatly affected by the conditions in which we experience it. It is amplified by stress and dulled by health and happiness.

Opioids for Acute Pain? A Qualified "Maybe." Opioids for Chronic Pain? Nah.

Opioids can be very effective for some types of acute pain (if you break your leg, narcotics can help) but they don't work well for chronic pain. Although opioids can help alleviate pain in the short term, with more prolonged use they end up rewiring the brain—to what degree and how quickly is highly individual. Over time, it takes higher doses to get the same effect. Lower doses bring on unpleasant symptoms of withdrawal, and also increased pain. So if you show up for your post-op check with your orthopedist asking for a refill on your Percocet, something is wrong—either with your surgically repaired broken leg, or with your relationship to your pain pills.

In keeping with that, the 2017 ACP guidelines do not recommend opioids for acute back pain and recommend them for chronic back pain *only as a last-ditch option*, after all other treatments have been thoroughly pursued and patient and doctor have had a serious conversation about the risks of chronic opioid use.

I think there are two situations in which one *could* consider *briefly* using opioids:

1. You're in so much pain you can't move (and you've tried everything else). You don't need to be doing human origami stretches, where you've folded yourself into a variety of interesting

configurations ("Look, I'm a swan!"), but you do need to keep moving. If you are frozen in bed or on the couch because you feel like your back is going to shatter like a rose dipped in liquid nitrogen, an opioid might get you moving again. But just one or two pills.

2. You can't sleep because of the pain. Sleep restores our entire body, not just our brain, so it's very hard to recover if the pain is so bad that it prevents one from sleeping. Of course, there are sleeping medications, and there are some older antidepressants that can help improve sleep and nerve pain. Try them first. But if it's the pain that's driving the insomnia, then a very, very occasional pain pill could help. But beware.

What about Surgery?

There are legions of books written about surgery for low back pain, including my seminal work, *OMG, Don't Do It!*, available on Amazon and also in eight boxes stored in the rafters of my garage.

Speaking of the garage, thinking about finally cleaning it out is something like contemplating surgical treatment of low back pain. The man cave may be a mess, and a pain, and highly dysfunctional (even though *everything* is *exactly* where it needs to be), but trying to address it will almost certainly be a lengthy and painful process. And before you pull the cars out and commit yourself to this monumental project, you need some assurances that the effort will be rewarded, that the New Garage Layout will be an improvement over the Old-But-Well-Established Garage Layout. Surgery is a big commitment: will it be worth it?

It depends on what kind of surgery you're talking about, and what the underlying back problem is.

Herniated Disc Causing Shooting Nerve Pain (Sciatica)

Multicenter studies show that 90 percent of those with sciatica will see their pain resolve in fewer than three months. If your sciatica is due to a herniated disc and you're developing significant leg weakness or the pain is so severe that you don't think you can wait three months, there is good evidence that performing a discectomy (where the surgeon removes the part of the disc that has herniated out and is pushing on a nerve) will speed the recovery. But a few months after the surgery, the folks who opted to wait for the herniation to crawl back into its hole are doing just as well as those who chose the scalpel.

A couple of notes: if a herniated or degenerated disc is believed to be causing low back pain but is not causing sciatica, results from a discectomy seem to be poor. And, a 'microdiscectomy' is generally a less invasive form of the standard discectomy.

Spinal Stenosis (Arthritis is Narrowing the Spine)

In the same way that arthritic knuckles can grow in size, arthritis in the spine can knuckle into the tunnels and pathways that nerves follow as they branch off the spinal cord, exit the spinal canal, and head out into the body. If one of the nerves heading down into the legs gets pinched by one of these "bone spurs," an Attack-o'-Sciatica can follow. Ideally, with a little time the pinched and swollen nerve usually returns to its normal size and the sciatica resolves.

If not, one may need to consider a surgical procedure called a "laminectomy," which entails removing the portion of the vertebrae (and the ligament running underneath it) that forms the roof of the pagoda that houses the spinal cord. This deroofing is designed to provide the spinal cord and exiting nerves with a little more wiggle room. For a year or two, this decompressive laminectomy improves pain and function better than supportive care, but thereafter the benefit is less apparent.

Disc Degeneration and Facet Arthrosis

The spongy discs that sit between the bony vertebrae of the spine degenerate as we grow older. They literally dry out and hold less water and the outer layer loses some of its rubbery toughness. Like a worn-out set of shocks on your car, when a disc is too shot to be a shock absorber for the spine, the ride gets rocky and pain follows. In some cases, the worn-out disc itself is the source of the chronic pain.

As mentioned earlier, each vertebra is connected to the vertebrae above and below it by a number of what are called "facet joints." Like

MAN OVERBOARD!

every other joint, if the cartilage lining and lubricating the facet joint starts to wear out, now you've got bone grinding against bone, and pain follows.

What to do about these two common spine problems? Here's where we get to what is arguably the most complicated and aggressive spine surgery: the fusion.

Spinal Fusion Surgery

Thankfully, a spinal fusion does *not* involve the use of weapons-grade plutonium, although you might feel that way immediately after the procedure. (I know a spine surgeon who sometimes warns his patients: "When you wake up, you're gonna hate me!")

In a fusion, the vertebrae above and below the problematic disc or facet joints are fused together using bone grafts (donated by bone from your pelvis or by a generous cadaver). Commonly, a couple of metal rods are screwed in place for additional support. That's right, screwed in place. Typically the spine is fused just in the back, along the spine of the spine (posterior fusion) but sometimes it will be fused from the front (anterior fusion) as well, and that's about as big as a spine surgery can get. Sometimes a badly diseased disc will be removed as well.

Theoretically, a fusion seems like a very definitive solution to low back pain. How can there be any more pain if the bad disc has been removed (or at least stabilized), the nerves and spinal cord are unpinched, and the fused joint can no longer move?

This theoretical definitive solution is a nice idea—and so is peace in the Middle East, and a fiber laxative that isn't so gritty. But once the spine is fused at one level, the mechanical stress is then borne by the vertebrae and discs immediately above and below the fusion, and it's unlikely they are showroom-new either. Perhaps that's why low back fusions tend to have short-term benefits that peter out to no-better-than-you-were over the long term, or why some patients eventually need to have additional levels surgically fused.

A 2009 review by the American Pain Society found only four high-quality trials using fusion to fix degenerative disc problems. Three of those found the fusion to have no better outcomes than intensive rehabilitation that included cognitive behavioral therapy—a type of therapy that helps patients with chronic pain (from any source) deal with the psychosocial factors that are contributing to their pain. The fourth study found fusion to be a better option, but only 16 percent reported an "excellent" outcome (no pain or restriction of function/movement) and less than half thought they had a "good" outcome (only sporadic pain, and slight restriction of function).

The strongest and clearest benefit for spinal fusion surgery comes if the spine is unstable due to the following:

a) scoliosis (a twisting of the spine)
b) spondylolisthesis, a condition where one vertebra has slid forward and out of its usual position in the spinal column, or
c) after a decompressive laminectomy surgery (see spinal stenosis, above).

Low Back Surgery: Where Big Money and Soft Science Collide

To be clear, I have nothing against short-term benefits. In fact, I am *for* them, hurrah! But every surgery carries operative risks, and the postoperative pain is probably going to be an 8.5 on the Richter scale. I have heard doctor skeptics suggest that the pain relief of low back surgery comes not from improved spinal mechanics, but from improved perspective, as in, "Now you know what intense back pain is *really* like!"

Low back surgeries are also incredibly expensive, which is to say lucrative for those performing them, or the folks who own the surgical suite. And the better something pays in medicine, the more it gets done—a "strictly business" setup that makes it feel like it's the business model reimbursement and not science that decides what works. A senior spine surgeon colleague of mine estimates that half of spine surgeries are unnecessary; and that half of the surgeries that are necessary are more aggressive and extensive than they need to be (e.g., performing a fusion when a simpler decompression will do; working on many vertebrae rather than just one).

But money also stokes competition and innovation, and there's plenty of that in the spine surgery world (by comparison, competition in the bedsore arena is very low). New devices and surgical techniques are being introduced at a steady pace, and maybe one of them will hit it big. In the meantime, the answer to excessive numbers of spine surgeries lies in making better decisions and fewer incisions.

The "soft science" part of the equation is that low back pain is difficult to study. Science is strongest when it has clearly measurable objective data: a cancer drug can be judged on whether it cures patients or prolongs lives, a heart drug on whether it prevents heart attacks.

Low back pain is defined by a uniquely personal and complex endpoint—pain—that is hard to standardize and measure. As noted earlier, we don't understand why some people can have a pretty beat-up looking spine on an MRI but report little to no pain or functional loss, while others have a fairly good-looking MRI but suffer from severe low back pain. Clinical trials for surgical treatment of low back pain are hard to do, because unlike a trial where the pill and the placebo look the same, surgical patients cannot be blind to, or objective about, the fact that they got randomized to have surgery rather than intense rehab. Although I presented three distinct scenarios for possible surgery (herniated discs, spinal stenosis, and degenerative discs/facet arthrosis), the fact is, patients often have a mix of these conditions that can be difficult to objectively measure or categorize for a clinical trial. Surgeons have standards of care, but they are not machines, and their techniques and skill levels vary.

I am not saying I would never have low back surgery, but I'd have to be at the end of my proverbial rope, having run out of patience, options, and Costco-sized Percocet PEZ dispensers. I'd want to be seen by a very thoughtful and cautious spine surgeon (they exist), and I'd want to know that my goals for surgery were aligned with what the surgeon felt could be achieved. Because I'd want to have some confidence that the garage remod was not going to degenerate back to a cryptically organized hellhole, which, by the way, is how Wikipedia defines the term *man cave*.

Warding Off Future Troubles

You read stories about a guy who owns a P-51 Mustang, the renowned World War II fighter plane, and hear that it takes about 500 maintenance hours to keep that bird airborne for an hour. From what I can see, the older one gets, the more maintenance work is required to remain physically active and vigorous without bunging yourself up and paying for it. There's little room now for the weekend warrior stuff you did in your 30s. You're not a World War II relic, but you're getting there.

If you've had significant back issues—either chronic, or more often than you'd like, or bad enough to scare you—then it's time to consider a low back maintenance program. A physical therapist can develop a more personalized and customized program, or you can find all kinds of suggestions on the Internet (choose a reputable source, of course). Whatever the specific exercise regimen, the idea is the same: maintain the strength and flexibility of the muscles, ligaments, and tendons that support your spine. And that includes your abdominal muscles. Remember, muscles play a *critical* role in converting a flexible spine into a rigid spine; if they get flabby, it's difficult for the spine to lock into its most supportive form, the one that will allow you to safely lift or carry a load.

Stronger core muscles will help you ward off future low back troubles, but so will a stronger brain. Here's how.

One of the unfortunate things about low back pain is that the spine doesn't typically give instant feedback. Ideally, it would say, *"Don't do that!"* and as long as you stopped doing "that," the pain would either never come, or instantly resolve. Disaster averted. But like a hangover, the punishment for an ill-advised low back contortion often doesn't arrive until the next morning. Sometimes it's even a day or two later.

Recognize this scenario? You help your daughter move a sleeper sofa into her new apartment. Admittedly, some of the ergonomics of getting up the back stairwell were a little wonky ("Are you sure this building is safe?" you ask her), but you made it. Everything was alright, alright, alright. Until the next day, when you reached for something low on a shelf and your back seized up like the crankcase had run dry. Suddenly you were not alright, alright, alright. Hardly.

When lifting things, use your brain to conscientiously follow good body mechanics. What this means is that you are displacing the weight (your own body weight, plus whatever you are lifting) down through the spine in the optimal way. The exact opposite of good mechanics is that demonic torture device, *the airport luggage carousel*. You CANNOT bend at the knees, so you're leaning out with a straight back; your spine is rotating and twisting as the bag moves past you; and the bag is too freakin' heavy. "Oh my God, what's in this thing!" you shout at your partner, who replies calmly and without a trace of irony, "I don't know. That's your bag."

"Bend at the knees!" is always good advice, but it takes more effort if your knees are starting to get stiff from arthritis.

Perhaps hardest of all, you'll have to begin recognizing when a task at hand—moving this over there, lifting that up to there—is maybe more than you should tackle. This confessional honesty will require that you either:

- Slow down (it can be done safely, but not as fast as you'd like)
- Figure out a better way (grab a dolly or your four-wheeler) or …
- Submit to the ultimate male humiliation: ask for help

THE SMOKER'S AMALGAMATED SINNER'S AND SERENITY PRAYER

Dear God,

I know that I am a smoker, and I ask for Your forgiveness.

I believe I will die from my cigarettes and wind up dead early.

And so I turn from my addiction to nicotine and invite You to come into my heart and mind, before they are clogged with atherosclerotic goo and I stroke out or have a whopper of a heart attack.

Grant me the courage to change these things—which *should be changed*, I agree—and the wisdom to distinguish between a chemical addiction and a bad habit, whichever one mine is, or both.

So that I can go on living one day at a time,

Enjoying one nicotine-free moment at a time,

Accepting the inevitable weight gain and hardships of withdrawal as a pathway to health,

As Jesus would have, if he had smoked, which he didn't. Not once.

Although he may have been tempted a time or two.

Amen.

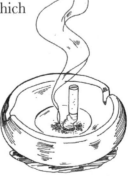

7 VICES

What were once vices are now habits.
—The Doobie Brothers

Smoking

Here's what a trove of lawyers, lobbyists, and a boatload of money can do for your cause in the good ol' USA.

In 1964, US Surgeon General Dr. Luther Terry released a seminal 387-page document on the hazards of smoking tobacco. Drawing from over 7,000 smoking-related articles, the report concluded that cigarette smoking caused lung and throat cancer in men, probably caused lung cancer in women, and was the single most important cause of chronic bronchitis (a common form of chronic obstructive pulmonary disease, or COPD). Since the release of Dr. Terry's landmark report, more than 20 million Americans have died prematurely of smoking-related illnesses, and yet this highly lethal and dangerous product remains legal.

Contrast this to the plight of the lowly "Jarts," those larger-than-life, lawn darts that many of us tossed around in the backyard as kids.

In 1988 the US Consumer Product Safety Commission imposed a nationwide ban on the sale of lawn darts, citing an unreasonable risk of death or serious injury. The ban included two exemptions: those lawn darts that didn't cause skull punctures, and "those products which, for sample (sic)

MAN OVERBOARD!

It's not "a bad habit," it's an addiction. It's the nicotine—a very powerful and very legal drug—that keeps you coming back, and it's the soot and carcinogens that give you heart and lung disease and cancer. If you smoke, quitting has to be Priority #1 on your health to-do list. Cold turkey vs. slow turkey? Everything works—just keep trying.

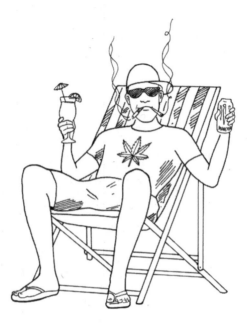

do not have pointed tips, are not intended to stick in the ground, and thus do not have potential to cause puncture wounds." And thus do not stick inside the yellow plastic rings that are the very basis of the game.

At the time of the Consumer Product Safety Commission's Jarts ban, that plastic-finned hellion of death had caused three fatalities in children and more than 6,000 injuries. Every death a tragedy, every injury unfortunate, but lawn darts banned, and cigarettes perfectly legal? Go figure.

Aren't We "Over" Smoking? I Thought Smoking Was Banned?

If you carry with you the nostalgic memory of coming home from a bowling alley, rock concert, or some other public event and peeling off your smoke-infused clothes before going inside, you might be under the impression that the fire of smoking is almost out. Hardly. Public smoking bans and strong persistent public health messaging have driven US smoking rates from 21 percent of adults in 2005 to 14 percent of adults in 2019. Three cheers and a couple of congested smoker coughs for a 7 percent drop! But if 14 percent seems higher than you expected, it might be because public smoking bans have also lowered our perception of how many people are still smoking, since most of it now occurs out of public view. But 34 million American adults are still at it, and according to the CDC, smoking rates remain highest in these groups:

- Men
- Adults ages 25 to 64
- People with a high school education or lower
- People living below the poverty level
- Midwesterners and Southerners
- The uninsured or Medicaid recipients
- Disabled people
- Those with a mental illess
- American Indians and Alaska Natives
- The LGBTQ community

It's Not a Bad Habit; It's an Addiction

You don't need to page through the surgeon general's report to know that smoking is unhealthy. This has been written into the human hard drive. We know this. When the smoke of the campfire genie spirals our way, we duck, we dodge, we fan it away. We don't sit there and deeply inhale. Smoke is, and always has been, an irritant to the respiratory tract, and getting out of the way is an ancient reflex arc.

What drug could possibly be powerful enough for us to ignore the primal message that smoke is to be avoided and not inhaled? Nicotine. It's as powerful as any addictive substance we know; it just happens to be legal. And that's why we do smokers a great disservice when we refer to smoking as "a bad habit," as if it were a matter of social etiquette. Changing lanes on the highway without signaling is a bad habit. Talking with your mouth full of food is a bad habit. But smokers don't have a bad habit; they have an addiction. Call it what it is. If you smoke, you are a nicotine addict. You tolerate the smoke to get to the nicotine.

There's not a smoker alive who doesn't know about the dangers of smoking (or using tobacco in other ways), but when I talk with patients about their addiction, they understandably like to counter with the few positive things they feel smoking does for them. "It calms me down" is probably the most common response, while the less introspective often say something like, "I don't know, Doc, I just like it."

But how could a brain stimulant like nicotine calm someone down? That doesn't make any sense—unless that person is withdrawing from it. The nicotine-addicted brain is having a love affair with this chemical, and when it's gone for too long, the brain gets ornery, fussy, irritated, anxious. The brain is shouting, "Where's my damn nicotine?!"

This is why a large national survey found that nearly one-third of smokers light up within five minutes of waking up, and nearly another third lights up between 6 and 30 minutes from wakeup. (This measure is such a good indicator of nicotine dependence that it has its own acronym TTFC, for "Time to First Cigarette.") Having not smoked since they dozed off hours ago, their brains wake up screaming for nicotine.

So remember this: once you're addicted to nicotine, you smoke to feel normal. That "calm place" that a cigarette brings you to is where everyone else (that is, the nonsmoker) lives. You like how you feel when you smoke because you don't like how you feel when you're not smoking. That's the essence of addiction.

Cold Turkeys and Warming Sleestaks

Kicking the nicotine addiction is like the childhood show *Land of the Lost*, wherein a father and his two children on a rafting trip accidentally plunge into the Cretaceous Period—a world of dinosaurs and low-budget special effects.

Whatever the plot line, each episode inevitably ends up in the deepest recesses of a cave just as the lizardy Sleestak monsters—cued by the final commercial break and/or plummeting nicotine blood levels—start to come out of hibernation. You can tell they're waking up because their big, beady red eyes start to glow, and they begin making clumsy, pawing movements at passersby. Nicotine withdrawal can feel that way.

There is one major decision to be made when quitting smoking: how do you like your turkey?

Going cold turkey means you're gonna abruptly stop smoking, and you'll fight the Sleestaks/nicotine withdrawal head-on, without medication. No dancing around, no looking for escape routes that will only disorient the film crew: just take them on, mano vs. lizardy bastard, until you've freed yourself from the cave. This is gonna hurt—the cravings, the irritability, the insomnia will last a week or three—but the directness of this approach brings a certain simplicity and clarity to quitting.

Going slow turkey means you're going to slowly cut back on the heaters, and try and sneak past the Sleestaks using stealth, diversion, and medications. The slow turkey/weaning approach makes the withdrawal process less arduous and intense, but it also makes it take longer.

These three types of medications that can help you fight through withdrawal:

Nicotine Replacement

The idea is simple: replace the nicotine you'd be getting from cigarettes with pharmaceutically grown nicotine (what are tobacco plants doing with all that nicotine anyway? Do they feel buzzed all the time?). At a minimum, you've eliminated all the carcinogens generated by burning tobacco leaves; and these take the edge off the nicotine withdrawal symptoms by providing you with nicotine.

Nicotine replacement comes in a variety of vectors: patches, gum, lozenges, nasal spray, and oral inhaler, but not as a pill or a suppository (thankfully). Most work similarly—except the patch, which releases a continuous level of nicotine in the blood. That's handy if you're a person with a very short and fierce TTFC. Because you're getting nicotine while you sleep, you don't wake up full-on gnarly Sleestak.

Bupropion (Wellbutrin, Zyban)

Antidepressants work by altering neurotransmitter levels in the brain, particularly those involved in our mood. One particular antidepressant, bupropion, seems to tone down the brain's response to nicotine withdrawal.

Varenicline (Chantix)

Varenicline binds to nicotine receptors in a way that produces a mild nicotine sensation but also blocks receptors from being stimulated by bona fide nicotine molecules.

Like all drugs, both bupropion and varenicline carry a list of potential but typically mundane side effects that I won't list here. But varenicline has a rather vivid one that's worth mentioning: it can lead to some very strange and even disturbing dreams. Some people even describe the horror of plunging into the Cretaceous Period on a cheap yellow raft, without the benefit of CGI.

Both of these drugs can be effective quitting tools, but there has been some controversy as to whether they can worsen underlying depression or other mental illness (which can happen *anytime* one is trying to quit smoking). Since smoking rates are significantly higher in those with mental illness, this particular side effect has been an important issue for these two drugs, important enough that it earned them a boxed warning from the FDA, counseling users to watch for serious changes in mood or behavior.

In the healthcare big picture, we regularly tolerate *serious* side effects and toxicity from drugs that treat *serious* conditions, say, cancer for example. A lot of chemotherapy drugs are what pharmacologists refer to as "nasty shit," but the situation requires them. And since smoking leads to more premature deaths than anything else, shouldn't we consider cutting varenicline and bupropion a little slack, or "Slee-slak"?

In late 2016, the FDA removed the boxed warning and issued a consensus statement noting that the mental health risks of these two drugs were lower than previously expected, rarely serious, and outweighed by the benefits of stopping smoking.

No Fumare. What Works Best—Cold or Slow?

In 2016, a British study found that people who went cold turkey had better cessation rates than those who went slow turkey. It may have something to do with resolve. In this study, those who indicated a pre-study preference for slowly reducing their cigarette use didn't do so well, suggesting that this preference was a tacit admission of not really being ready to quit—"I'd prefer to take this slow." But note that people

MAN OVERBOARD!

successfully quit in both groups. How many times you try to quit might be more important than how you try to quit.

Call for Help—You'll Do Better

There is conflicting evidence on whether prescription medications like bupropion or varenicline are more powerful than nicotine replacement therapy. There is also some contradictory evidence regarding whether the benefits of these three medications seen in clinical trials really hold up in the "real world." There are a lot of possible explanations for noted differences, but one might be that clinical trials require smokers to plug in to a support group. They get instructions on how to use the medications correctly. They know that someone out there is rooting for them.

What everyone agrees on is that interventions like behavioral therapy and counseling improve quit rates by helping smokers address the psychological and behavioral struggles of addiction. You *can* do it alone, but you're not likely to do it as well.

Which leads us to the gold standard for stopping smoking: combining medication and behavioral therapy. They both work, and they work better together.

Will I Get Fat?

There are all kinds of amusing and interesting excuses for not quitting, and weight gain is high on the list. Nicotine is a mild appetite suppressant and a stimulant—both of which tend to suppress weight gain. It is well known among smokers that quitting smoking can lead to mild weight gain. This issue has been studied in detail, and the news is good: the health benefits of not smoking definitely outweigh the health risks of gaining a few extra pounds.

How about E-Cigarettes?

E-cigarettes, those battery-powered cigarette droids that vaporize (hence the term "vaping") a concoction of nicotine, propylene glycol and various flavorant chemicals, were initially promoted as cancer-sticks-without-the-cancer, but there is increasing evidence that vaping can lead to significant lung injury, and carcinogens have been found in some e-cigarette products. Further research is needed, but for now, it's probably reasonable to think of e-cigs as a *somewhat* less unhealthy form of the unhealthy behavior of smoking. Can e-cigs help someone quit smoking? The CDC's "bottom line" is that current research doesn't provide a clear answer to that question, although there are some studies showing that the use of e-cigs containing nicotine are associated with higher cessation rates compared to using e-cigs without nicotine. Given that, why not stick with the many other safe, effective, and scientifically-proven nicotine replacement options?

Every Attempt Brings You Closer to Quitting

A 2015 survey found that although 55 percent of smokers had attempted to quit in the previous year, only 7 percent were successful in quitting. It's hard to see failure as a success, but each failure makes you smarter and more familiar with the nooks and crannies of your personal addiction. Schedule a quit day. Tell everyone who cares. And try and try again.

Alcohol

The piano has been drinking not me, not me, not me
—*Tom Waits, "The Piano Has Been Drinking (Not Me)"*

MAN OVERBOARD! Excessive drinking includes binge drinking, heavy drinking, or drinking while pregnant or underage. Binge drinking is by far the biggest problem and leads to nearly half of all alcohol-related deaths, i.e., being intoxicated is VERY unhealthy. What defines alcoholism? Not being able to stop despite serious health and personal life consequences. Cirrhosis develops in 10-20% of excessive drinkers, and typically requires a decade or more of drinking. The antioxidants found in wine will not protect you from the wrath of its alcohol.

Alcohol is like gambling in that the majority of people can enjoy either of them responsibly. Unfortunately, for a small fraction of the population, the relationship is ruinous.

The public image of an alcoholic is the homeless, staggering drunk, but on the surface at least, the lives of most alcoholics appear surprisingly normal. They do all the regular life things and sober up as best they can for the serious parts. They drink a six-pack on lunch break (think about the sheer volume involved!) and keep a low profile for the first few hours back at the office. It takes a lot of skill and grit to be a functioning alcoholic (as most alcoholics are). You have to be able to lie and mislead people, particularly those who are closest to you—unless you married a fellow alcoholic, and then you're home free. Sort of.

It can be difficult to know how much alcohol is too much alcohol. Working at a hospital, I ask every patient I am admitting how much and how often they drink. The answer might not have anything to do with why they need to be in the hospital, but alcohol withdrawal carries a big head of physiologic steam, and if you don't start treating early, it can get ahead of you. Quite commonly, the amount they admit to drinking starts out low on the first day of admission and then steadily rises through their stay. It can be hard to be honest about one's true drinking habits.

The CDC's National Center for Chronic Disease Prevention and Health Promotion defines four subcategories of "excessive alcohol use":

- Binge drinking
- Heavy drinking
- Drinking while pregnant
- Underage drinking

What'll It Take?

Let's begin by clarifying what constitutes a "drink." The answer is 14 grams of alcohol, which is helpful if you're a scientist, or maybe a bartender. For the rest of us, a drink is 12 ounces of regular beer (~5 percent alcohol content), 5 ounces of wine (~12 percent alcohol), or 1.5 ounces of distilled spirits (~40 percent alcohol).

Binge drinking for men is defined as five or more drinks in a couple hours; for women, it's four drinks. In both cases, that should be enough to push their blood alcohol concentration past the legal driving limit of 0.08 g/dL. Heavy drinking is defined as 15 drinks a week for a man, and 8 for a woman.

As a CDC infographic emphatically trumpets, "Binge Drinking is the Main Problem." Not only does it include 90% of excessive drinkers (one in six Americans binge drinks, tossing back an *average* of eight drinks an average of four times a month), but binge drinking is also far more likely to leave one drunk and dangerous. Being intoxicated is acutely unhealthy. The intoxicated die—and kill—in car crashes. They choke on their own vomit, fall down stairs, get into fights, have unprotected sex, damage their unborn child. When one looks at cause-of-death statistics, it's a major player in the category titled "Unintentional Injury." So it's no surprise that binge drinking leads to about half of the deaths and three-quarters of the costs of excessive alcohol use.

Who binge drinks? It's twice as common in men, but it's not just frat house stuff. It peaks in the 25- to 34-year-old age group and doesn't really fizzle out until the retirement years. The percentage of binge drinkers is higher in people with higher incomes, but the smaller percentage of binge drinkers in lower income groups tend to have more frequent and furious benders. Binge drinking is fairly consistent across different education levels, and is more common in the Midwest.

Too Much of a Good Thing: When Does "Social Drinking" Become "Alcoholism"?

As if binge drinking doesn't have enough detractors, bingers are more likely to develop what is now termed alcohol use disorder (an umbrella term that includes alcohol dependence, alcohol abuse, alcohol addiction and the colloquial alcoholism). A 2014 CDC study found that 10% of binge drinkers could be characterized as having an alcohol use disorder, compared to 1.3% for the rest of those in the excessive use category (heavy, pregnant, underage).

Although it's easy to quantify or objectify how many ounces of alcohol are in a standard drink, and how many of those drinks will get an average person officially intoxicated, it's more difficult to decide who *exactly* has an alcohol use disorder. The standard general definition is someone who cannot stop or control their drinking despite the fact that the booze is starting to give them serious health problems or turn their personal and work lives into a dumpster fire

That's a logical approach, but there are some problems in using those criteria as benchmarks.

Serious Alcohol-Related Health Problems Often Show Up Seriously Late

If you don't kill or injure yourself while intoxicated, the short-term health effects of drinking are typically transient and rarely serious (a bad bout of hepatitis or pancreatitis being an exception). They are often easily dismissed. "See, I'm fine now. What's the problem?"

The serious, long-term health effects of drinking—primarily liver disease and neurologic damage to the brain—are not as easily dismissed. Some 10-20% of those who drink excessively will develop liver cirrhosis, but it typically takes a decade or more of hard drinking before that happens.

There's a fair amount of diversity in how resistant some drinkers are to the physiologic damage of alcohol, just as there is for smoking. We don't understand very well why, pack for pack, some smokers get emphysema and others don't. Or why some very heavy drinkers don't develop cirrhosis, while some drinking less excessively do. It would be nice if we could give each person a clear boundary—"You drink this much over this many years and you will get cirrhosis"—but that's not how it works. There are a few lab tests that can point to heavier alcohol intake, and sometimes a stiff bout of alcoholic liver poisoning ("hepatitis") can give an alcoholic an early warning. But too often, the symptoms from the most definitive findings of alcoholism—the cirrhosis, the brain changes—come too late to make any serious course corrections.

I've diagnosed end-stage cirrhosis in a few retirees who lived—quite successfully, thank you—through the three-martini luncheons of the *Mad Men* era of business, and then continued the festivities with a couple of vodka sours at happy hour through their retirement years. They certainly didn't consider themselves to be alcoholics, and they took their new diagnosis of alcoholic cirrhosis as a slap across the face, an affront worthy of a pistol duel. But their alcohol-saturated livers were looking for an early retirement.

One Man's Dumpster Fire Is Another Man's Regular Dumpster

I'm a doctor, not a judge or a marriage counselor, but with some regularity I am asked to referee a conversation between family and patient, where the family wants to (understandably) use the seriousness of the hospital setting to finally confront their father/mother/sister/brother about their alcoholism.

The argument commonly starts with a rousing discussion about how much the patient is actually drinking. Sometimes this involves counting bottles or cans in the recycling, or trips to the liquor store. Often the patient feels that the family is seeing double ("I don't drink half of what they say I do!").

Eventually the conversation turns to how much of a problem his or her drinking has become. You know how this goes: the family describes a social or work-related dumpster fire, and the alcoholic goes on a long diatribe about how everyone is misinterpreting the flames, and if there is a problem, it's because people are making too much of the fact that he likes to have a few drinks now and then. If they stopped pestering him, maybe he wouldn't drink so much. Denial and deception are part of alcohol use disorder, and they can tear a family apart. As a bystander, the details aren't that important; what's important is that the alcoholic is being confronted with his disease and its consequences. That is the beginning of progress.

A diagnosis of alcohol use disorder can be hard to quantify, and the diagnosis isn't taken lightly, so medical professionals like to get it right. A book called Diagnostic and Statistical Manual of Mental Disorders has a list of situations designed to ferret out the severity of a person's alcohol abuse:

- Continued drinking in spite of deteriorating relationships with family and co-workers
- Going to great pains to not be without alcohol
- It takes longer to physically recover from a bout of drinking
- Withdrawal symptoms (such as headache, nausea, sweating, insomnia, tremors)
- Increasing symptoms of anxiety or depression

Of course, the criteria have to be answered honestly, which an alcoholic in denial is not likely to do.

I can say this: if you're arguing with your spouse or kids about how much you drink, you do have an alcohol problem. You may not have boarded the Coors Light Silver Bullet, but you're hanging around the station.

Wine Will Get You There

When I was growing up in the blue-collar super-boonies of Chicagoland, only the winos drank wine, and we didn't know any winos. Of course, that all changed with the Two-Buck Chuck revolution, which made wine more accessible. But just because your ethanol comes all dolled up in fancy grape juice doesn't mean you can't be an alcoholic. My wife and I had lost track of a bubbly, vivacious friend of ours: and when we ran into her years later, she announced, to our great surprise, that she had finally conquered her alcoholism. She was a great cook, we knew that, but it turned out that a good portion of the wine she was cooking with didn't end up in the food. She loved to cook in part because it was the perfect cover for her alcoholism. More often than not, the wino is in the kitchen, or in the study, or watching Netflix, and not out in the gutter.

Red wine has long been touted for its medicinal effects, in part because the French—despite their rich diet and historical fondness of smoking— seem to enjoy exceptional health. Red wine contains antioxidants and the best known one is resveratrol. In animal studies, resveratrol seems to have all kinds of health benefits, but the doses required were large. To replicate this with our diet, humans would have to eat either 7 kg of peanuts, or 2500 kg of apples, or 2.8 kg of dark chocolate, or drink a minimum of

500 L of red wine *every day*. The dark chocolate is tempting, but the red wine dosing would be lethal. The best advice I've ever heard on the subject came from a cardiology colleague of mine, who told his patients, "If you like a glass with dinner, fine. But don't use wine as medicine."

Caffeine

I've seen the light, oh the light I've seen, I've seen the light of St. Caffeine.
—*John Gorka, "St. Caffeine"*

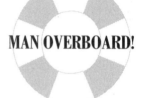

Caffeine is not a vice, it's a healthy elixir! And that's due to all the health-promoting antioxidants found in coffee beans and tea leaves. Conversely, caffeinated sugar-soaked carbonated beverages are a nutrient desert, and energy drinks get their "energy" from veterinary doses of caffeine. Avoid both unless malnutrition is your thing, or you're looking to hop on your skateboard and pull a 360 Ollie heelflip.

Given its ancient and ubiquitous nature, no drug has been more widely "tested" in humans than caffeine. If it had any of the serious consequences that tobacco does, we'd know about them by now.

Caffeine is a stimulant, just like nicotine, but the benefits of the caffeine in coffee and tea have to do with the company that caffeine keeps. Nicotine hangs around with a litany of biochemical thugs, the ones that cause cancer and atherosclerosis. Conversely, the caffeine in coffee beans and tea leaves associates with a number of biochemical nuns—antioxidants that run around the bloodstream doing God's work, with the occasional rap across the knuckles with a ruler for bad behavior. The caffeine in energy drinks and carbonated beverages has been synthetically derived, not brewed, so imbibers are missing out on the good stuff.

The primary "energy" boost in energy drinks is high-dose caffeine, but they may contain other stimulants as well, and miscellaneous vitamins, amino acids, and minerals are typically thrown in to confuse the consumer and substantiate the monster price. Beyond synthetic caffeine, all carbonated beverages can offer is grams upon grams of sugar. Similarly, adulterating your coffee with industrial doses of caramel brûlée syrup and whipped cream might be good for your taste buds, but the personal health benefits will have been diluted.

Because we consider caffeine to be such a friendly drug, used in such a friendly way by friendly people, we tend to overlook the fact that it can be addictive. Granted, a caffeine addiction will not leave you flat broke and toothless like a meth addiction, but you can get hooked. Drive by a Starbucks early in the morning, and there might be a line of caffeine junkies circling the block, waiting for their hit of caffeine. Some of them are feeling pretty darn ornery, and that's because their brains have been without caffeine overnight. I wonder what their TTFC—Time to First Caffeine—is.

Common symptoms of caffeine withdrawal can include fatigue, irritability, depression, anxiety, problems concentrating, and headaches. With some regularity I will take care of a caffeine addict who's just gone through surgery and can't eat. They're getting as-needed doses of intravenous narcotics, so you'd think they'd be feeling little pain of any kind, and yet they complain of a booming headache. The hammering quickly dissipates when you can finally get some sips of coffee into them and they're visited by Our Lady of Hope and Vigilance, Saint Caffeine.

Most of us recognize what it feels like to be too caffeinated—jumpy, fidgety, wired up. And because caffeine raises our heart rate in the same way that adrenaline does, it's logical to think that an espresso might make the heart a little jittery, leading to energetic heart beats that we call "palpitations." (People often describe their palpitations as "having skipped a beat." That feeling can be due to extra beats being added to the normal cadence, or more powerful contractions of the heart.)

That logic thread makes so much sense that 80 percent of US doctors recommend that patients with palpitations or other heart dysrhythmias either abstain from or limit their caffeine intake. And yet a 2018 State-of-the-Art Review by the American College of Cardiology concluded otherwise: "Although there is no clearly defined threshold for caffeine harm, a regular intake of up to 300 mg/day [~3 cups of coffee] appears to be safe and may even be protective against heart rhythm disorders." Yes, *protective*.

The review included three additional caveats:

- If you have clear personal experience of caffeine making your heart flutter, then cutting back makes sense.
- Energy drinks are a different animal: they tend to have much higher amounts of caffeine and contain other energy-boosting stimulants that can trigger dysrhythmias. The analysis is complicated by the fact that energy drink users are more prone to mix them with other drugs.
- And the best caveat of all, particularly if you wear a St. Caffeine pendant around your neck: Large studies have found that regular caffeine imbibers have lower cardiovascular and overall mortality.

One caffeine buzzkill deserves mention: if it's messing with your sleep, and it certainly can, then any health benefits are lost. Most sources recommend stopping caffeine a minimum of six hours prior to bedtime, but the number is personal. For some, lunch is the cutoff; for others it's dinner.

Marijuana

But let me get to the point, let's roll another joint
—Tom Petty, "You Don't Know How It Feels"

MAN OVERBOARD!

Like caffeine, THC has a long and relatively safe track record with adult, non-pregnant Homo sapiens. But this is not your grandpa's marijuana: potency rates are rising quickly, which could transform this drug into something we don't recognize. Doesn't seem to cause lung cancer but can cause chronic bronchitis. If you have an aching desire to try marijuana but wouldn't dare, give cannabidiol (CBD) oil a try. It can't hurt, and it just might not help.

Marijuana (aka reefer, pot, grass, weed, Mary Jane/MJ) has long been America's most popular illicit drug, and legalized medical and/or recreational use in an increasing number of states has increased its public profile if not its usage.

The active ingredient in marijuana is tetrahydrocannabinol (THC). After entering the blood stream, THC quickly binds to cannabinol receptors. Believe it or not, all of us—even those of us who would only identify a roach as an insect—have reefer receptors! These receptors are part of a complex network of nerves deep in the brain that regulate movement, coordination, learning, memory, and higher cognitive functions such as judgment. They also spark senses of pleasure and reward. Even a tokeless brain makes its own cannabinoid molecules to run this operating system, so smoking MJ just hyperactivates a pre-existing natural system.

It's THC's ability to stage-dive into the reward centers of the brain that brings the characteristic "high" of the drug, as well as a relaxed feeling. Depending on the user, some might also feel an altered perception of time, a heightened sensory perception, the archetypal munchies, or the kind of laughter canonized by Cheech and Chong.

Those are the good things, the buy-in, but there are a number of bad things too, like diminished short-term memory (musician David Crosby tweeted, "If smoking marijuana causes short-term memory loss, what does smoking marijuana do?"). Higher doses can induce a paranoid, psychotic reaction, and long-term use can bring on schizophrenia in certain susceptible patients. Even after the THC has left the system, problems with sleep and memory can persist, sometimes permanently.

While the acute effects of THC are mostly independent of age, THC use clearly interferes with the development of the younger brain, so that heavy use in teens can result in permanent cognitive processing delays. The developed adult brain is less sensitive, but heavy marijuana use can still lead to a list of psychosocial problems that'll put you at the top of the guest list for the *Dr. Phil* show:

- Lower life satisfaction
- Relationship problems
- Work issues including absenteeism, accidents, and increased propensity to job-hop

This Isn't Your Grandparents' Marijuana

Like caffeine, marijuana (THC) is a drug that has been tested in humans for thousands of years—except that the marijuana of today is not the marijuana of our ancestors. In the early 1990s, average THC levels were lower than 4 percent. By 2018 they had climbed above 18 percent. And not only have we put our green thumbs to work cultivating plant varieties that produce more THC, we've also figured out how to "distill" THC oils so that they are much more potent, with THC concentrations of 40 percent to 60 percent (or higher).

How unhealthy are these new-and-"improved" forms of marijuana? As with social media and addictive Internet games, this is a large, unsupervised social science experiment whose outcomes may not be understood for years. As noted above, we know that higher doses of THC are more likely to bring on the more "psychotic" effects of the drug—anxiety, agitation, paranoia, psychosis. But we don't yet understand how these more potent versions will interact with the developing brains of teens and young adults. And since these more potent forms are generally vaporized and inhaled, we don't understand how toxic they will be to the lungs (some of what is being vaped or vaporized is residual solvent from the distilling process).

Weed Warriors: THC behind the Wheel

A 2013–2014 survey by the National Highway Traffic Safety Administration (NHTSA) found that 12.6 percent of weekend nighttime drivers tested positive for marijuana, a nearly 50 percent increase from a study done in 2007.

Well, that can't be good. There's ample laboratory data showing that THC impairs a number of important driving-related skills such as attention, judgment, coordination, reaction time, car following, speed control, and the ability to perform evasive emergency maneuvers. Despite all of that weed in the driver-performance garden, studies have been mixed on whether impairments measured in the lab setting actually mean anything on the road.

In 2015, the NHTSA published the results of the most definitive study yet on the crash risk involved with marijuana and other drugs.

On the face of it, THC use seemed to increase the risk of being involved in a crash by 25 percent. But when researchers accounted for other risky-driver features—men have a higher crash rate than women, younger drivers crash more often than older drivers—the use of THC didn't seem to have any effect on crash risk. It appears that higher-risk drivers are the ones most likely to smoke marijuana, and that doing so didn't increase their risk further. *Dude!* The study took place in Virginia Beach, where marijuana use was illegal at the time. The obvious question is whether legalization in states like Colorado will alter that crash risk data by increasing either overall THC usage or individuals' THC drug levels.

CBD Oil: Try It on Pancakes

CBD oil seems to fit all the criteria for a medical fad. Everyone is selling it, sales are skyrocketing, but no one knows exactly what it's for. "If it doesn't work, then why is everyone buying it?" seems to be the kind of primitive group-think psychology that continues to drive sales. Like some Prohibition-era drugstore "cough syrup," we are led to believe it works for everything, and its association with THC gives it the titillating allure of being nearly illegal. A little clandestine.

CBD stands for "cannabidiol." Behind THC, it's the second most common cannabinoid in marijuana, but it doesn't seem to generate any of the pleasurable "high" feelings that THC does. What we do know is that it has a good safety profile, and that there doesn't seem to be any addiction or abuse potential.

The FDA has approved Epidiolex, a pure form of CBD, for use in children with severe, treatment-resistant seizure disorders. Beyond that, the therapeutic uses for CBD are mostly speculative and theoretical. A 2017 report from the World Health Organization lists 17 diseases/symptoms for which CBD *may have* therapeutic benefits, including "suppression of nausea and conditioned gaping in rats." (As best I can tell, scientists use rats—who cannot vomit but can "conditionally gape"—to assess whether a new medication is likely to induce nausea.)

Don't get me wrong: I'm hoping that CBD oil will cure everything from cancer to kookamunga fever, but I'll wait for more research to roll in. Trouble is, from a historical perspective, an industry that is piling up profits selling an unproven product has little incentive to bankroll studies that might prove it doesn't work. What's the upside to *that*?

Is Smoking Marijuana Physically Unhealthy?

It seems like the unhealthy effects of smoking marijuana are mainly confined to the brain and the lungs. One would think marijuana smoke, which is so dense that it can penetrate reinforced steel and also any garment worn to a rock concert, would be likely to increase the risk of lung cancer. But so far the evidence is inconclusive. It can, however, lead to a chronic bronchitis similar to what cigarette smokers develop. As I mentioned earlier, one really needs to train the lungs to accept super-heated noxious gases, and even then, they don't like it.

THC can be addictive—about 9 percent of those who use marijuana will become dependent on it, and they'll feel awful when they try to stop, just like nicotine addicts.

I know adults who are daily users of marijuana and think of it as their form of yoga or meditation: a time to relax and elevate the mind. They seem to be fine. They are not looking for derision or approval. If it somehow relaxes them to the point where they lose the urge to text while driving, it might even save their lives, not shorten them. Even so, since THC seems to stimulate the same reward areas of the brain as sex and chocolate, it might make more sense to stick with the safer options of sex and chocolate, particularly dark chocolate, which contains antioxidants and cannot lead to pregnancy. As far as we know.

8 SLEEP

Sleep, Sleep, the Magical Deal, the More You Sleep— the Better You Feel

The often-heard advice "You can sleep when you're dead" exudes a sense of industry, personal resolve, and even gratitude: *We only have one life to live, so let's make the most of it!*

But personal experience—and better yet, modern sleep science—tells us we won't make the most of our lives if we are sleep deprived. Unless your goal is to lead an ornery, fatigued, depressed, achy, listless life, with a Golden Gate–caliber mental fog and the frazzled emotional control of a preschooler. Then, yes, absolutely. Stick with it.

Sleeping is not laziness, and it's not optional, no more than emptying your bladder or bowel is. And sleeping is not a passive act. Although we might look like we're dead, we are very much alive when we're sleeping, as the brain and body are actively being rebooted.

Sleeping is restoration. Not that we understand exactly *how* that restoration works. Of all our organs, the

MAN OVERBOARD!

Sleep is the overnight battery charge our brain and body need. Miss out and get messed up. Seven to eight hours per night ought to do it. Start with good sleep habits: douse the lights; bedroom cold, quiet, and dark; bed for sex and sleep only; go to bed tired (exercise); avoid heavy meals, alcohol, and caffeine; same time every night, even weekends. Sleeping pills better short-term option than long-term. Cognitive behavioral therapy can put you to sleep. Obesity epidemic has made obstructive sleep apnea much more common. Insomnia symptoms and snoring followed by pause in breathing, then gagging and sputtering are classic symptoms and will buy you a sleep study to prove it. If so, a CPAP mask will likely be a nighttime companion.

brain is arguably the most complicated and mysterious. The heart is a pump, squeezing out blood. The kidneys filter blood, reabsorb the good stuff and let the bad stuff drain into the whiz bucket. The skin keeps our insides in.

But the brain? How does a network of nerves, firing in a particular pattern, create a thought or an emotion, or vividly rebroadcast a memory? And why do we need to sleep? To attempt some answers, let's start with the basics: the factory settings.

An Ancient Ritual

Sleep is an ancient ritual, like having sex or dunking breakfast items into coffee. And for that reason, it's controlled by the deeper and older ("primitive"? Hardly!) parts of our brain that are sometimes referred to as our "lizard brain" (but not by lizards, of course). The newer, top part of our brain, the cerebrum ("gray matter," "cerebral cortex") handles the more complicated stuff: memory, complex thoughts, voluntary movements, sensations, emotions, perceptions.

Because humans are diurnal (daytime creatures) our brain must synchronize the sunnier segments of our circadian rhythms with our lights-out sleep rhythms. Circadian rhythms, controlled by our brain, hormonal system, and autonomic (automatic) nervous system, optimize our physiology for what the day requires of us: becoming physically active, shoving food down the pie hole, answering endless emails, dressing from the waist up for Zoom meetings, texting the kids (who appear to be perpetually occupied with other, more riveting texts from people who definitely did not bring them into the world).

Command control for sleep lies in a number of areas of the brain, including the hypothalamus, an (unshelled) peanut-sized area near the base of the brain. It houses the opulently named "suprachiasmatic nucleus," which takes information it gets from the retina on current light levels and relays it to the brain's pineal gland, which makes melatonin, a neurohormone that helps tuck the body in for sleep. All tissues—not just the brain—have receptors for melatonin and it would be nice if just taking a slug of it could put us to sleep, *naturally*. But, as with so many other things in medicine, it is a whole lot more complicated than that, because taking melatonin as a sleeping aid is only mildly helpful.

Sleep Cycling: Rinse and Repeat

If you believe Robert Dean Lurie's *Begin the Begin*, a book about the quintessential 80s and 90s band R.E.M., you're probably aware that the band's moniker stands for Ralph Eugene Meatyard, an optician and photographer from Kentucky who signed his prints "REM" and whom frontman Michael Stipe admired. Seriously. This is a much more intriguing and, frankly, Stipe-like story than the more common and bourgeois explanation, that Stipe stumbled onto "rapid eye movement" while scouring the dictionary for lyrics.

Sticking with the more precise, scientific nomenclature, sleep can be divided up into the Ralph Eugene Meatyard (REM) phase, and the non–Ralph Eugene Meatyard (non-REM) phase. Because the Meatyard estate is notoriously litigious and defensive of Ralph's legacy, I will use REM and non-REM from here on out.

Each night, we move between REM and non-REM sleep, with each cycle lasting about 90 minutes and then repeating four to six times in an evening. Here's what's happening:

REM Sleep

REM doesn't start until about 90 minutes into sleep. When it does, our eyes dart back and forth behind closed eyelids, and our brain-wave activity moves toward wakefulness. Although one can dream anytime during sleep, REM dreams are the most vivid. Thankfully, during REM our arm and leg muscles are temporarily turned "off" so we don't hurt ourselves by acting out our dreams. (We know what that looks like, from all the memes showing people injuring themselves flailing away with their virtual-reality headset on.)

Why do we dream? Why is there a "w" in "swordfish" when "sord-fish" would do? We spend about two hours per night dreaming in la-la land, but we can't recall most of it—thank goodness. If, as some speculate, dreams help us process the emotions and events of the day, then the clarification must be happening at a deeply subconscious level. Because I don't see how my wife giving birth to a very large hamster, with Krusty the Clown as midwife, as a tornado rips through the neighborhood and the ice cream man (who looks suspiciously like a med school classmate) refuses to break a $20 bill...really, I don't see how that clarifies anything. In fact, I can't recall ever having had a clarifying dream.

Non-REM Sleep

Non-REM sleep has three stages.

- Stage 1 lasts just a few minutes; as the body physically relaxes and slows down, brain activity slides out of wakefulness and into a drowsy state.
- Stage 2 is considered light sleep, which means it has half the calories and just 10 percent of the flavor of regular sleep.
- Stage 3 is deep sleep, the most restorative and refreshing stage. And yet, this is also the stage when sleepwalking occurs, typically one to two hours after falling asleep. It's most common in childhood and ends in the teen years. I selflessly entertained my family with various sleepwalking exploits, except for the time I tripped and smashed my mouth on the clothes hamper. This Stage 3 deep sleep typically occurs earlier in the night.

What Does Sleep Do for Us?

From an evolutionary point of view, sleeping doesn't make a lot of sense. Instead of gathering food, building empires, fornicating, or putting together the quintessential alt-rock band of the '80s and '90s, we're lying there helpless, oblivious to the world and therefore vulnerable to it. There must be a big payoff for all that risk.

For both the brain and the physical body, sleep is a time to repair, to haul away biochemical debris from the day and restock the shelves. The 86 billion neurons in our brain are richly interconnected through what are called "synapses." During sleep, some of these synapses get scaled down, pruned back. Not all of the synaptic "connections" we make during the day ("that barista is wearing a funny hat") are worth keeping. If you keep writing on a whiteboard and never erase anything, it won't take long before you'll be out of space. A hard drive that is too full works slowly. Not only do we throw stuff out during sleep, we also file things away, taking the information we learned and collating it with what we already know ("I know who would love a goofy hat like that; isn't her birthday coming up?").

This filing process makes it easier to find and remember things, and it can also make new connections for us. In that way, the "passivity" of sleep becomes both creative and productive. Writers commonly recall waking up in the morning to find that a passage they were struggling with the day before seemed to have "written itself" overnight.

How Much Sleep Do We Need?

A consensus statement from the American Academy of Sleep Medicine and the Sleep Research Society recommends that adults should get seven or more hours of sleep per night, on a regular basis. More than nine hours on a regular basis might be appropriate for young adults, people recovering from sleep debts, or those dealing with illness.

Yes, we all know somebody who seems to get by—very successfully—with very little sleep. And the reason is genetics, and perhaps a Lifetime Achievement Award from Caribou Coffee. The exception should not prove the rule, however, and the rule is: sleep deprivation is bad for us. Sometimes it's dangerous. "Microsleep" describes the several-second bursts of daytime sleep that the chronically sleep deprived sometimes experience. Marked by head bobbing, eye drooping, and momentary lapse of concentration, when microsleep happens behind the wheel of a car, it can be macrodeadly. The National Highway Traffic Safety Administraton reported that in 2017, drowsy driving led to 91,000 crashes and nearly 800 deaths. Since drowsiness is harder to test for and objectify (compared to a breath test for alcohol), those numbers are likely an underestimate. When it comes to driving, wake up, America!

Snoozology: Insomnia and Obstructive Sleep Apnea

There are a number of categories of sleep disorders, but insomnia and sleep-related breathing problems are by far the most common. Insomnia comes in three basic flavors:

- Difficulty falling asleep (takes more than 30 minutes)
- Difficulty staying asleep
- Waking up too early

About one-fifth of adults experience short-term insomnia (lasting up to three months) and 10 percent suffer from chronic insomnia (occurring at least three times a week for at least three months).

Insomnia doesn't typically pop up all on its own. Usually there is something triggering it, and often the trigger is obvious:

- Stress (you've heard others speak of this)
- Medical problems, particularly chronic back pain or arthritis
- Pregnancy (only the appetite improves "with child"; virtually everything else suffers)
- Menopause (that burning smell is the scorched sheets)
- Alcohol (you might doze off quicker with a nightcap but you'll probably wake up not long after)
- Caffeine (if you need an explanation, you've never tried caffeine)
- Environmental factors such as a snoring bed partner, or a cheap hotel room, or being homeless
- Lifestyle issues (night-shift or swing-shift work is a common cause, but anything that makes it hard to stick to a regular sleep schedule will do it)
- Medications (most often mental health medications, because they work through the brain)

MAN OVERBOARD!

Insomnia and mental health issues such as depression and anxiety are common problems that are commonly interrelated. One can lead to the other.

Sleep Like a Baby (Let's Stay Positive!) with These Healthy Habits

Don't Mess with Your Pineal Gland

Bright lights in the evening mess with your pineal gland, which secretes the sleeper hormone melatonin as the darkness of night sets in. Blue light is a particularly potent suppressor of melatonin, and although it is a portion of all light (natural or bulbed), there is a lot more of it coming from electronic device screens and LED lighting. Avoid bright lights and blue light for two to three hours before bed, and if that just ain't gonna work for you, get a blue light filter or some blue-blocking glasses. Red light is easier on the pineal gland, so a dim, red night light is a good option that will give your bedroom an edgy brothel feel.

Avoid These Things in the Evening

When the sun calls it a day, stay away from alcohol, caffeine, nicotine, and heavy meals. Your brain complains, "You had all day to eat, why now?"

Create Sacred Sleep Space

The bedroom should be quiet, dark, and cool. Expectations are everything: use your bed exclusively for sleep and sex, so that your brain knows what to expect when you slide between the sheets. Work from the kitchen table or the sofa. Watch TV somewhere else.

Exercise Regularly

Being physically tired does wonders for sleep. You'll have to figure out for yourself how close to bedtime you can safely exercise. For many, evening exercise provides an energy boost that makes it hard to doze off.

Make a Routine of Your Routine

Go to bed and get up in the morning at roughly the same time every day, even on weekends and during vacation.

Momentum Matters!

Don't go to bed if you don't feel sleepy (a good routine could prevent this problem).

If you don't fall asleep after 20 minutes, get up and don't come back to bed until you feel tired.

Avoid naps, particularly long ones or late ones. They reduce your sleep momentum at night.

Don't Escalate. Tone It Down.

Time to exchange the Rage Against the Machine or Foo Fighters for some Townes Van Zandt or the soundtrack to *Interstellar* (unless you're prone to weird space-travel dreams). Relax. You can balance the checkbook or argue with the kids in the morning. And get rid of the bedside clock. You're awake. Getting upset about what time it is will not help you fall back asleep. Just the opposite.

"What Next? Can't Drugs Help? Why Won't You Give Me Drugs?"

Let's say you've successfully implemented everything on the Good Sleep Habits list but still struggle with insomnia. What's next?

Of course, everyone's heard of sleeping pills, which historically have been some kind of sedative. Like alcohol, those drugs helped people nod off, but that doesn't mean they could produce meaningful restorative sleep. People in the ICU are often heavily sedated, and when we bring them out of what is commonly referred to as a "drug-induced coma," they certainly don't feel mentally refreshed and rested.

The sleeping pills of yore were addictive and dangerous (think: overdose) and commonly caused daytime somnolence—which some then treated with stimulants. This sometimes led to a vicious, dangerous cycle of needing escalating amounts of sedatives to sleep, and then escalating amounts of stimulants to wake up. Till they woke up dead.

Today's sleep aids—Ambien being the most widely recognized—are more refined but still have side effects, including sedation and clouded thinking. They are not addictive in the sense that going without them will cause signs of physical withdrawal, such as sweating, fast heart rate, and agitation. But if you take them regularly, you might find that you can't sleep without them, and then you're "hooked."

By the way, most over-the-counter sleep aids contain diphenhydramine (Benadryl) as the active ingredient. It's an antihistamine with sedating properties, as anyone with allergies knows.

Best "Drug" for Chronic Insomnia Isn't a Drug

The drug of choice for chronic insomnia is not a drug, but rather a psychological treatment called "cognitive behavioral therapy" (CBT). As the name implies, one meets with a therapist to try and root out (and then change) the thinking patterns or learned behaviors that have kept you from conquering insomnia. (Why count sheep if sheep make you nervous *and* you have a wool allergy?)

Ruminating thoughts and anxieties that were drowned out by the busyness of the day can sometimes grab center stage when we go to bed. Certain thoughts can lead to other certain thoughts, thereby escalating our anxiety. CBT can help recognize and eliminate these dysfunctional thought loops, so that you end up somewhere different than staring at the ceiling. You may learn relaxation techniques as well.

The ultimate goal of CBT is to acquire the skills needed to be one's own therapist, so that you can make your own adjustments in your mental golf swing.

Sleep Apnea

Ask anyone with a new baby in the house: interrupted sleep is bad sleep. Sleep is meant to be one long symphony, no intermissions or potty breaks, no disruptions.

One of the most common interrupters of sleep is obstructive sleep apnea (OSA). As noted earlier (if you hadn't dozed off), when we fall asleep, our muscles relax. That includes the tissues in the back of the throat and the neck, and the tongue. If these relax enough, they can begin to block the airway (that's the "obstruct" in "obstructive sleep apnea"), preventing adequate airflow in and out of the lungs. Subsequently, oxygen levels fall and carbon dioxide levels rise until they reach a critical point that triggers the respiratory centers deep in the brain to begin yelling, "Wake up and breathe!"

If you've ever had the slightly nerve-wracking privilege of watching someone go through spells of sleep apnea, you'll see the breathing get slower and shallower until it stops ("apnea" means "not breathing"). Then, when the brain's apnea alarm goes off, they begin to gasp and snort and sputter, and their breathing catches up by getting bigger and faster.

Although apnea sufferers don't typically wake up during an apneic period, they are roused from deep sleep back to light sleep, where they have to restart the process back to deep sleep. The more apneic spells, the more Z's lost. This explains why people with obstructive sleep apnea wake up in the morning feeling like they never went to sleep, unlike those with insomnia (who can tell you exactly how long it took to finally fall asleep, or that the clock read 4:15 a.m. when they woke up for good). Patients with sleep apnea can't explain their daytime exhaustion. Not only does sleep apnea lead to B-movie zombie traits, the poor breathing can lead to medical problems such as heart disease, high blood pressure, heart failure, and stroke.

For obvious reasons, many people with sleep apnea snore, but not everyone who snores has apnea. Snoring followed by a silent breathing pause, then gasping or choking, is a stronger indicator of sleep apnea. Similarly, most people with sleep apnea are shaped like Skipper and not Gilligan, but not every obese person has sleep apnea, and skinny people can develop it too (I imagine an episode where the Professor makes a CPAP machine out of coconuts and bamboo). Sleep apnea is more common in men, and in those with a larger neck size (16 inches for women and 17 inches for men). It also tends to run in the family—perhaps because of inherited traits like neck length, jaw shape, and body size.

There are self-assessment screening tools you can fill out online to see if you're at risk for OSA, and they are all set up to have high sensitivity—that is, they don't miss many cases of OSA. Depending on how you answer the questions, you might need to visit a sleep doctor and then get a confirmatory test. Those come in two flavors.

Overnight Sleep Study

An overnight sleep study is performed in a sleep lab, where you will be hooked up to a dazzling array of sensors, including some that will record your brain waves, heart and muscle activity, oxygen levels, and astrological karma fluctuations. Off go the lights, and you're free to fall asleep and do your thing: snore loudly. If, over the course of the evening, the technicians monitoring the process definitively conclude that you have OSA, they'll fit you with a CPAP (Continuous Positive Airway Pressure) mask and then adjust the settings to make sure it's working optimally. Sleep labs and CPAP masks are generally managed by pulmonologists—lung doctors—who will see you in follow-up.

As the name suggests, most sleep studies are done at night, except for swing-shift or night-shift workers, where daytime testing is a more realistic reenactment of their sleep habits. And sleep labs are set up to evaluate the entire gamut of sleep disorders, not just OSA.

Home Sleep Apnea Testing

Overnight sleep studies are spendy, but so are CPAP machines, and so historically speaking, insurance companies wouldn't pay for the mask unless you had a lab-based sleep study proving you to be deserving of the honor. But just like Zoom killed the commute, technology is changing things. If your doctor thinks it's likely you have sleep apnea, and you don't have a lot of other serious medical issues—particularly heart or lung problems—your doctor can arrange for you to have a more basic sleep apnea test that can be performed at home.

Unlike testing in a sleep lab, home monitoring can detect only sleep apnea (not other sleep disorders), but if it does confirm sleep apnea, you'll get set up with a CPAP mask and be on your way. Sweet dreams.

NUTRITION: HOW WE WENT CUCKOO FOR COCOA PUFFS

The Low-Fat Craze Left Us Gobbling Down Carbs, and Fatter Than Ever

As a certified healthcare professional, I want to relay to you, the lay reader, the entire breadth and depth of the nutritional knowledge I've acquired through years of medical training. It goes like this:

People need to eat.

People eat by putting food in their pie hole, aka mouth.

If a person can't eat via the pie hole, a tube can be threaded down into the stomach so that they can be fed that way.

If it's impossible to slide a feeding tube down into their stomach, the tube can also be put in surgically through the abdominal wall. If that doesn't work, intravenous feedings can be used.

When people eat too much, they get fat. When they don't eat enough, they get skinny.

People should eat in a "balanced way," with some of this and some of that, but not too much of "this" at the expense of

MAN OVERBOARD!

Low-fat mania had us demonizing all fats, but plant oils are healthy, except coconut and palm oil. Animal fats are less healthy, except cold-water fish. Trans fats are terrible ("Please, do *not* pass the margarine"). Instead, avoid simple sugars, and choose complex carbs. For protein, go nuts!— and beans, eggs, and lean meats. Fruits and vegetables are perennial powerhouses.

"that," or they'll end up imbalanced, and that's not good. What we're shooting for is balance.

There you go: that's everything I learned about nutrition in seven years of medical school and residency training. It also dovetailed nicely with what I learned from my high school health teacher (who was also the wrestling coach, although I didn't wrestle). He was a good guy, but his chain-smoking habits made him a somewhat less-than-credible candidate for the job. We never *saw* him smoke, but his clothes exhaled like a bowling alley of yore, and he had the kind of voice that suggested his vocal cords had been charred beyond recognition by too many heaters. He was not the picture of health, but he taught it. The class itself was only slightly more complicated than driver's ed.

What I think I remember him saying was something about how the crafty Egyptians erected the first food pyramids, way back in the Way-Back Period. This made a deep impression on me, particularly when you think of how healthy the ancient Egyptians look as depicted in hieroglyphs. Very svelte. Very slender. Very healthy.

From high school health to medical school, the subliminal message was that nutrition wasn't an important part of health—*if it was, we'd spend more time on it, you idiot!* (Is it possible to be yelled at subliminally?) That view is supported by the National Board Exams, the series of tests that any board-certified doctor must pass. Those are tests that are generally devoid of any questions about human nutrition but do have a lot of detailed questions about medical esoterica such as parasitic conditions you might see if you're working in an Urgent Care in, let's say, central Senegal. But not anywhere else.

Armed with this woeful lack of nutrition knowledge, doctors have two choices. The first would be to recognize that you—the all-knowing, but really not-knowing, doctor—are backed up deep in your own territory. Time to bring out the punter. Simply tell the patient, "You're overweight. You don't eat right. Would you like to see a dietician?"

Duck as you say this because they might get mad, and when you return to a standing position, try to explain: "Listen, if this were a rare case of schistosomiasis, or hobglobulin fever, I might be able to help you, but you're just obese, and so you're on your own." If the patients recock their arms or just bristle at something dismissive-sounding in your tone, throw them a bone by having clinic staff print them a copy of the Egyptian food pyramids. Scribble a reminder across the top: "Remember to eat a balanced diet."

The second option for the nutritionally malnourished doctor is to educate him- or herself on the subject, and this is what I chose. Encouraging me was the embarrassment of having a partner who knew more about nutrition than all of the diplomates of the American Board of Medical Specialties combined.

So I studied up, and I've been following the public health messaging (much of it driven by private interests) on how to "eat right" long enough to watch it careen back and forth like a drunk riding on a unicycle.

There's a lot to know, but there's even more that we don't know, so you can make this as complicated and confusing as you'd like. One way to avoid excess calories is to make every meal into something like a SpaceX rocket launch, with thousands of checklists and double checks and looks of consternation, so that by the time you're finally ready for launch—time to eat!—the stress of the preparation has killed your appetite. This is an effective approach, but it's not a lot of fun, particularly if you enjoy eating.

So although the science of nutrition is constantly evolving and endlessly complex, I will try to make this SPS (Simplification for Purposes of Sanity) simple. One *can* cut corners if the corners don't really count.

How We Went Cuckoo for Cocoa Puffs

Let's start our dietary journey with a historical perspective.

Having defeated the Nazis and the Imperial Japanese in World War II, America set out to destroy its toughest enemy: itself. It was a three-pronged attack designed to bring the human body to its arthritic knees.

Rising affluence meant that everyone could afford to smoke, and smoking seemed to be the real A-bomb for human health, scorching blood vessels into atherosclerotic ash and causing cancer by leaving genes looking like bent and twisted pieces of metal. Everyone seemed

to be smoking, including doctors, who, rather notoriously, were sometimes used in tobacco endorsement ads ("Give your throat a vacation...
Smoke a FRESH cigarette," says the young surgeon, who's holding a
pack of Camels instead of a scalpel). It was 20 years before US Surgeon General Luther Terry released the first federal government report linking smoking and ill health, including lung cancer and heart
disease. But by 1964, we were hooked. Many remain so: 14 percent of
adult Americans still smoke.

The second prong in our attack on good health, "Operation Pie
Hole," aimed to fundamentally change food—how much and what
kind. The mechanization of farming and cheap energy drove food
prices down into the root cellar; and although that still didn't wipe out
hunger, it did make calories abundant and cheap. It was a super-sized,
high-fructose-corn-syrup revolution that made us fatter than ever, and
rising obesity rates made diabetes a household name.

It wasn't just the quantity of food that changed, it was the quality.
A rising industrial food complex promised to liberate women from
their kitchens and gardens by developing processed foods, canned
foods, and foods with the shelf life of Shakespeare. The convenience
of prepared foods was indeed liberating to women, but nutrition was
lost in the bargain. Sodium and sugar became the bedrock "spices"
of prepared food. Flavorants lied to our tongues, twisting the time-
worn axiom "If it tastes good, it is good" so much that a food scientist
could make your shoes taste like a peach. None of the nutrition of
the peach, but yum!

The third prong of the attack was physical convenience. All labor
could be considered menial and be avoided. The automobile replaced
the dog as man's best friend. A leisurely life was a good life, and a
perpetual cavalcade of labor-saving devices came to rescue us from
the banality of physical movement: escalators, electronic toothbrush-
es, elevators, leaf blowers, and, God be praised, the drive-up window.
Since obesity is kind of a cash-in, cash-out ledger, the convenience of
modern life made us cash heavy, adding to the obesity and diabetic ep-
idemics and eventually giving rise to nationwide chains of forced labor
camps with names like "LA Fitness," "Bally Total Fitness," "Chunky
Earl's Incomplete Fitness."

Big deal. You've got all-natural meats sliced by hand. I've got turkey and ham, made by science.

—*Tony Bolognavitch, the King of Cold Cuts, Jimmy John's sandwich commercials*

The Scarlet "F," as in "Fat"

By the 1960s, several decades of dedicated smoking were adding up to increasing rates of heart disease. Smoking seemed to increase the risk considerably, but the underlying problem was atherosclerosis—fatty buildup inside the blood vessels that was either narrowing them or closing them off completely. And so it made sense to avoid fats, not only because they seemed to cause atherosclerosis but also because at 9 kcals per gram, fat was far "richer" and calorically dense than protein or carbohydrates (4 kcals per gram).

In an era when we discovered that the moon was made of moon dust, not cheese, we also firmly and logically concluded that it was fat that was making us fatter. Only one of those ideas would hold up over time.

And then the Inuits and the Greeks came to our rescue! What do those two geographically distant groups have in common, other than oceanfront views? Low rates of cardiovascular disease and diets high in unsaturated fats. The increasingly beloved Mediterranean diet is heavy in healthy olive oil, which is monounsaturated, and the oil in cold-water fish is also unsaturated.

There are two basic kinds of fats: saturated fats and unsaturated fats—chemical terms that indicate how many hydrogen molecules are attached to the carbon frame of the fat molecule. Saturated fats seem to be more prone to stimulating atherosclerosis, and unsaturated fats seem to fight against it. Try to remember, "Sat fat bad, sat fat bad," although that's a bit hyperbolic. Saturated fats are not Jim Jones Kool-Aid; they're not going to kill you. It's just that in most cases, unsaturated fats are the healthier options.

How to keep all this fat talk straight? Animal fats tend to be less healthy fats and are often solid at room temperature. Plant fats tend to be healthier and are typically liquid at room temperature. There are a couple of exceptions to this animal-fat-worse, plant-fat-better rule. Fish oils are high in omega-3 fatty acids, a family of health-promoting polyunsaturated fats. Because our bodies require but can't make omega-3 fats, we have to get them from our food. Since cold-water fish such as salmon, lake trout, herring, sardines, and tuna tend to have the most omega-3 fatty acids, the Inuits derive more benefit from their locally caught fish than do the Greeks fishing in the bathwater of the Mediterranean. But let's see the Inuits try to raise olives.

The other exception to the "Animal fat is less healthy" rule is wild game, which doesn't contain a lot of fat to begin with, and what it does have is mostly unsaturated. The lesson here is that when you domesticate an animal, restrict its activity, and give it access to unlimited calories (sound familiar, humans?), it gets fat, and more of that fat is saturated. This also explains why grass-fed meat has a healthier fat profile.

The two exceptions to the health-promoting effects of plant oils are coconut and palm oil, both of which have high concentrations of saturated fats. In another triumph of marketing over science, coconut oil has been elevated by some to superfood status, despite the fact that it is wallowing in sat fat (87 percent, versus 63 percent for butter and 40 percent for beef fat), and despite the fact that a 2020 editorial in the American Heart Association's *Circulation* magazine labeled it "one of the most deleterious cooking oils." That was gut-wrenching news to people like me who enjoy eating a spectacularly tasty Thai dish that's lathered in it. Some experts advise putting coconut oil in the ice cream category—a tasty treat—but come on, who puts ice cream on stir-fried vegetables?

As the above percentages point out, all oils are a mix of several different types of fats: even the very healthful safflower oil has some small amount of saturated fat in it, and coconut has some unsaturated fat.

And one last fat fact: the trans fats found in partially hydrogenated oils are unhealthy. Evil Food Scientists of the 60s (a grunge band from Seattle) discovered that when they hydrogenated plant oils, the shelf life increased and the oils were more stable when subjected to heating. The last part is key, because hot oil is a critical ingredient to our national pastime, fast food.

The best-known partially hydrogenated oil is margarine, which at some point deposed butter as the grease of choice on rolls, pancakes, and potatoes. Only years later, we discovered that butter is the healthier option after all, and that trans fats are more powerful promoters of heart disease than saturated fats.

In 2006 the FDA opted to publicly humiliate trans fats by requiring that they be listed on food labels. In 2015, the FDA declared trans fats to be no longer GRAS (Generally Recognized as Safe) and announced a phaseout through January 2020. So long, sweet margarine. Hello butter, and also "butter substitute" made out of safflowers and salmon parts and recycled newspapers.

Fat Factoids
Plant fats are better because they're primarily unsaturated, except palm oil and coconut oil. Animal fats are less healthy because they're primarily saturated, except cold-water fish and wild game. Trans fats (partially hydrogenated oils) are *really* bad.

The Low-Fat Craze Sent Us Scurrying for Sugar and Salt

Since it made sense that too much fat was making us fatter than ever, Betty Crocker and her secret squeeze, the Pillsbury Doughboy, went to work lavishing the public with all kinds of low-fat goodie options. The major hurdle in getting to the utopian fat-free world was taste. Fat tastes good; it's satiating and imparts a fullness and richness to food. If these fat-free options were going to taste different from the packaging they were enclosed in, there was little option other than to replace the fat with the tried-and-tested salt and sugar.

Let's compare three versions of a popular ranch dressing. You'll see that as the fat goes down, the sodium, carbohydrates, and sugars go up.

Original: Fat 14 gm, sodium 260 mg, carbs 2 gm, sugars 1 gm, calories 130
Light: Fat 5 gm, sodium 310 mg, carbs 4 gm, sugars 1 gm, calories 60
Fat-free: Fat 0 gm, sodium 320 mg, carbs 6 gm, sugars 3 gm, calories 30

Shenanigans like this distracted the audience from a few realities:

- Robbed of the fat flavor, salad-goers were more likely to dump several servings of dressing on their salad in a desperate attempt to get it to taste like something more than pasture clippings. Or, they'd eat more of something else.
- It turns out you can get fat by eating low-fat cookies, particularly if you have to eat the entire box to feel satiated.
- In the food industry, if you're short on flavor, pile on the salt. And excess sodium is not healthy.

Fat-free is not a great option if the fats you're turning down are healthy ones, i.e., you're replacing a plant oil–based salad dressing with a fat-free/high-sodium/high-sugar option. Calorie for calorie, olive oil is healthier than sugar.

Cotton Candy, Alpine Turds, and the Glycemic Index

So low-fat mania pushed the dietary needle away from fat and toward carbohydrates, the simplest of which is sugar, and the needle on the nation's weight scale just kept going up. But the "low-fat blues" eventually forced us to take a better look at carbohydrates, which are essentially various complexes of sugars. It turns out that all carbohydrates are not created equal, and metabolically speaking, cotton candy is a much different carbohydrate than a whole-wheat roll.

As carbohydrates are digested and absorbed, they enter the bloodstream as glucose, and a surge of insulin is released by the pancreas in order to transport those glucose molecules into key tissues such as muscle and liver. The term "glycemic index" was designed to give consumers a more objective sense of how quickly a particular carbohydrate enters the bloodstream as glucose.

White bread has a very high glycemic index—you can have your jaw wired shut and shove a wad into your cheek like a plug of chewing tobacco and digest it just fine. On the other hand, an "alpine turd whole-wheat roll" from your local Earthy food store might take hours to chew and swallow and be absorbed (which is consistent with your finding that, on cross-section, the roll looks remarkably similar to a Duraflame log). Portions of the alpine turd might never be absorbed, which is an extra benefit for colon health.

Since food is fuel that we quite literally burn (oxidize), you can think of it this way: high-glycemic-index foods burn like paper towels—a flash of heat and then it's gone. A soft wood such as pine makes a nice, hot fire but it won't last the night. But a low-glycemic-index wood such as oak releases its energy and heat nice and slowly.

Why does the glycemic index matter? Isn't a calorie a calorie, no matter how quickly or slowly it's burned? There isn't a perfect answer for that, but we do know that the "hot fires" that sugars ignite are not healthy. Sudden, steep rises in blood sugar levels bring similar steep rises in insulin secretion, and high insulin levels aren't good. They trigger inflammation, and inflammation is the spark igniting bad physiology, including atherosclerosis and arthritis. The steep insulin spikes eventually lead to steep falls in insulin levels, and those sudden sharp declines seem to trigger hunger sensations. This is why, two hours after you scrounged a candy bar out of the back of your desk drawer at work ("Thank God, I'm starving!"), you find yourself hungry again. Simple sugars simply aren't satiating. A bowl of granola will get you all the way to lunch, but Count Chocula or Cocoa Puffs will desert you by 10:30.

It's easy to find glycemic-index lists for a whole array of foods, but for the sake of ease, forget about the list and just keep this in mind: the more "predigested" a carbohydrate is, the higher the glycemic index. Instant oatmeal, for example, has been predigested by the rollers at the Quaker oats plant, whereas the old-fashioned version has been chewed on a lot less. Native Americans did not harvest Minute Rice into their canoes. Wild rice needs chewing.

There are two exceptions to keep in mind: pasta is a highly processed form of wheat, but the way it's glued together makes it harder to digest and lowers its glycemic index (and whole-wheat pasta is better for you than regular pasta). Potatoes aren't processed at all of course, but believe it or not, their starchiness gives them a higher glycemic index than table sugar. This is bad news to a nation in love with French fries, but that news is tempered by the fact that fat tends to lower the glycemic index of any food, seeing as it slows absorption. And that's why ice cream (good ice cream, with a high fat content) has a lower glycemic index than one would think.

Interestingly, sugary, highly refined carbohydrates appear to be so unhealthy that they've given a deceptive twist to some studies reporting no association between dietary saturated fat intake and cardiovascular disease. What these studies tell us is that if you remove saturated fats from your diet and replace them with sugars or other refined carbohydrates such as white bread or instant oatmeal, you've done little to improve your health or your cardiovascular risk. The switch will push your bad cholesterol (LDL) down, but your good cholesterol (HDL) will go down too, so that the trade is neutral healthwise. If you're obese or inactive, the swap for carbs could worsen your insulin resistance, making the trade an even worse idea.

Carbohydrate factoids

Low-fat diets sent us scurrying for low-fat, high-sugar, and high-salt options.

Highly refined, high-glycemic-index carbohydrates wreak havoc with insulin levels and cause inflammation—and end up making us fatter than ever. Oh, and the extra salt might drive our blood pressure up.

Swapping saturated fats for sugars and highly refined carbohydrates backfired.

Fruits and Vegetables Weather the Storm—Go Nuts! and Beans and Eggs

Although fat was demonized (and then partially redeemed), and highly refined carbohydrates and sugars are in the doghouse, fruits and vegetables have remained above the fray. They continue to pack a powerful nutritional punch, with high levels of vitamins and minerals (some more than others), low levels of sugar (some lower than others), and healthy, slow-burning complex carbohydrates (yes, some more than others). It's as if we were born to eat these things, which we were. What's not to love?

Some people love protein, particularly strict carnivores. It's the third major molecular component of food, and it's every bit as important as carbohydrates and fats. We have to have it.

When it comes to animal proteins, it's important to keep in mind what kind of company the meat keeps: does it have a lot of saturated fat mixed in with it? It's also important to recognize that we've been bamboozled by the beef industry to believe that protein = meat, and that we are what we eat: if you want muscle, you better eat meat.

What the cattle or poultry industry will not tell us is to "Go Nuts." And yet that's a great idea: nuts are a fantastic source of protein and contain health-promoting unsaturated fats and oils. Beans are another great source of protein, and eggs, once vilified for their cholesterol content, are now recognized as a healthful, affordable, easily accessed protein source.

Udder Confusion: Dairy Foods Caught in the Low-Fat Crossfire

"I see you're drinking one percent. Is that 'cuz you think you're fat? 'Cuz you're not. You could be drinking whole if you wanted to."
—Napoleon Dynamite, referring to Deb's milk

A walk down the dairy aisle at Whole Paycheck Foods suggests that food scientists have now figured out how to make "milk" out of everything except recycled tires. Oat milk, soy milk, almond milk, milk of magnesia.

Some of the demand for the nondairy milk alternatives is likely because of milk allergies and veganism. But the bovine industry was hit hard by low-saturated-fat recommendations that put dairy foods and their naturally endowed saturated fats nearly on a dietary "no fly" list. Low-fat milk and yogurt could be tolerated, but only as a good source of calcium (also available in other common foods) and vitamin D (not there naturally: the dairy, not the cow, added it).

Then the Prospective Urban Rural Epidemiology (PURE) study came around 2017 and threw everything into udder confusion. Researchers looked at the intake of milk, yogurt, and cheese in 136,000 adults from 21 lower- and middle-income countries on five continents. (They were going to include butter, but there was so little consumption of it that they couldn't draw any conclusions.)

Researchers found that during the nine years of the study, those who had more than two servings of dairy per day, compared to those who had none, had a 16 percent reduction in the composite risk of death, heart attack, heart failure, and stroke. In fact, when each of these four disease categories was looked at individually, higher dairy intake was associated with a benefit in each disease category except heart attack—where the risk remained the same. The benefit associated with increased dairy intake was the strongest in stroke, which was reduced by 34 percent.

Though the study was indeed PURE, it was not perfect. (What dietary study ever is? It is difficult to control—or even just record—what people are eating over any meaningful period of time.) But the results of the PURE study begs the question, "When we 'Got Milk?' what do we got?"

Milk is mostly water, but it also contains lactose, calcium, and protein—32 to 34 grams per liter of it, with 80 percent of that being casein (a major ingredient in the production of cheese curds), and 20 percent of it being whey. It has milk fats, of course, but 60 percent of them are monounsaturated, polyunsaturated fatty acids, and medium-chain saturated fats, all of which seem to have different, and *healthy*, metabolic actions. The remaining 40 percent of milk fats are saturated, the kind we have traditionally thought of as promoting atherosclerosis.

But traditions are changing. A 2016 "authoritative review" in the American Heart Association's flagship magazine *Circulation* cited new evidence showing that saturated fats with an odd number of carbon molecules in their chain are health-promoting, while even-chained saturated fats tend to be unhealthy.

And here's the kicker: the unhealthy even-chained saturated fats in our bodies are primarily synthesized by the liver in response to increased dietary intake of carbohydrates and alcohol. Whereas the healthy odd-chained saturated fats come primarily from our diet. To an ice cream fiend, this is welcome news. Please pass the whipped cream! I am trying to ward off a stroke.

Check, Please

The low-fat craze and the obesity epidemic that followed has been a boon to the diet industry, and to every magazine, newspaper, or media outlet that wanted to trumpet the Next Big Thing in weight loss.

This perpetual blizzard of media coverage blurred the lines between "diet," as in trying to lose weight, and "diet," as in what should we be eating. I will talk more about diet plans and weight loss later in the book, but this chapter is about nutrition—finding the best food fuels to keep our bodies running well.

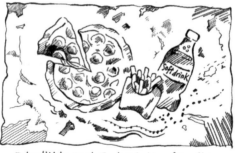

Paleolithic Fast Food painting from the Lascaux caves

Whatever the specifics, the paleo diet asks a very important question: what were humans designed to eat? There is no evidence that our paleo ancestors subsisted on French fries and beverages sweetened with high-fructose porn syrup (you read it right: this stuff is food porn). Before the arrival of agriculture, humans' food was diverse by necessity—a truly progressive dinner spent roaming the countryside for seasonal vegetables, nuts, berries, and roots, and supplemented by the lean meat of wild game. The advent of farming and grain production increased carbohydrate production, but none of the grains were processed (predigested) in any way similar to today. (When I was a kid, we brought home some pancake mix milled at a "Pioneer Village" we visited; it took steady resolve and several weeks to chew our way through a three-pound bag of sawdust pancakes. They made Bisquick pancakes seem like angel food cake.)

If humans were engineered to run on diesel, today's highly processed, predigested, sugar-soaked foods are like high-octane dragster fuel. Even our fruits and vegetables have been selected for increasing sweetness and less fiber.

All that said, it's not that complicated. You can have your fun—go ahead, have your pizza and your Lucky Charms. You just can't subsist on them.

What we all need to eat is good food, healthy food, real food. Michael Pollan, a prophetic voice in nutrition, recommends not eating anything your great-great-great-grandmother wouldn't recognize as food. "Eat food, not food products," he advises.

The counterrevolution of food has begun. Betty Crocker is overweight and bone tired, and the Pillsbury Doughboy is out on medical leave. What's good for us dietarily has always been good for us. Lemon Jell-O is not a lemon. As Pollan's books point out so expertly, when it comes to nutrition, we're heading back to the future.

10 SUPER-SIZED NATION
Amid a National Obesity Epidemic, Finding the Real You

Like comb-overs and chain-link fences, fat jokes are thankfully becoming a thing of the past. Fat is not funny. Chris Farley was fat and funny, but the core of his comedy was the contrast between his obesity and his incredible athleticism and alacrity. He was a gifted physical comedian, despite—or, in some ways, because of—his girth.

Overweight people have the misfortune of dealing with a private health issue that is publicly visible. One can smoke in solitude, for instance, but one cannot be overweight only in private. They don't need to be shamed or pointed out. Progressive Insurance is running a series of ads with "Dr. Rick," a life coach who helps homeowners who are becoming their parents. He is standing in a big box store with a few of his clients when a man with blue hair walks past them. Dr. Rick repeats calmly and clearly: "We all see it. We all see it," buuuuuuuut, his clients blurt it out anyway: "He's got blue hair!"

Unfortunately, when it comes to obesity "we all see it, we all see it" too much. Here in the United States we're experiencing an epidemic of obesity, with roughly a third of Americans being overweight, and another

MAN OVERBOARD!

Extra weight is unhealthy. A beer belly is more dangerous than thunder thighs. BMI adjusts weight for height, but can't tell fat from muscle. Don't "diet"—instead, change the way you eat. Avoid processed carbs and sugars. There's no weight-loss nirvana—find your own path. Exercise is always healthy, but a 25-minute workout can easily be erased by a grande latte.

third who are obese. Other countries that have embraced our version of modernity are seeing the same trends.

I've done medical work in poor, rural areas of South and Central America, where everyone is lean by necessity (limited calories) and circumstance (life demands physical work). So when the exceedingly rare overweight patient comes in and you ask the interpreter, in essence, "Hey, who's this heavy-set guy?" the reply is almost always something like, "He's the mayor." In other words, he's connected—both to money *and* calories—and he doesn't do much manual labor.

Here in the United States, we have a lot of "mayors." That's not good.

Obesity! What Is It Good For? Absolutely Nothing, Say It Again. Obesity! What Is It...

We often think of excess weight primarily as a cosmetic issue, though studies show that Americans are finding flab less unattractive and more flabulous than we used to. Diet ads on TV focus exclusively on the before-and-after look, and never feature one of their clients proclaiming, "I took 10 points off my blood pressure!" Looks don't kill, but obesity does, sending many to an early XXL grave.

Being obese contributes to poor health in myriad ways. It's as if it is unnatural, which it is. Wild animals don't become obese unless their environment (winter, cold ocean temperatures) demands it. You don't see an eagle that weighs 75 pounds, or a squirrel weighing 15.

Metabolically speaking, excess fat distorts our normal physiology. Like Axel Foley stuffing a banana into a Beverly Hills cop's tailpipe, things just don't run right. We've got a name for it: metabolic syndrome. Too much body fat causes insulin levels to rise, leading to diabetes; blood pressure rises into the hypertensive range; and the levels of unhealthy fats in our blood ratio ("cholesterol levels") also rise. All three of these things—diabetes, hypertension, and hyperlipidemia—are major promoters of the arterial inflammation and scarring ("atherosclerosis") that causes strokes and heart attacks. In the *Star Wars* saga, the wildly corpulent Jabba the Hutt's end came as he was choked to death by the chains of the fetching and scantily clad

Princess Leia, which, all in all, is not the worst way to go. But here on Earth, if you're overweight and human, it's usually a heart attack or stroke that gets you.

As if strokes and heart attacks aren't bad enough, obesity is a risk factor for a number of cancers, and it appears to be the primary driver in nonalcoholic fatty liver disease (NAFLD)—an excess of fat deposition in the liver. NAFLD can sometimes lead to Non-Alcoholic Steatohepatitis, which can cause cirrhosis (liver failure). Since NAFLD is now the most common cause of liver disease worldwide, it will likely become the most common cause of cirrhosis, ahead of alcohol and viral liver infections.

Topping things off, our country's obesity epidemic has led to an epidemic of sleep deprivation due to obstructive sleep apnea. Excess weight is a major risk factor for obstructive sleep apnea, a condition where intermittent periods of diminished breathing leave patients waking up feeling dead tired, even though it seems like they slept the whole night through. You can read more about it in the Sleep chapter.

So you read it here first—excess weight is unhealthy. The only conceivable benefit would be a hedge against hypothermia, or if you're preparing to hibernate, or if you wanted to have a chance to be the first contestant on *Naked and Afraid* who didn't have to entertain the audience by stumbling around buck naked in the wild groveling for food. You could just swat flies in your makeshift shelter, burning off the stored calories while waiting for the producers to raise the white flag.

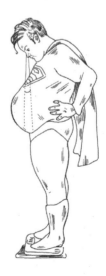

Body Mass Index (BMI): Adjusting Weight for Height

Your bathroom scale can tell you how much you weigh, but it can't tell you if you're overweight. The most common way to figure that out is to calculate your body mass index (BMI), which divides one's weight in kilograms by the square of one's height in meters.

(Somehow, America—the world's technology leader—just couldn't figure out the metric system, and now we're paying for it.)

The BMI works on the principle that there is a requisite amount of weight for any particular height, i.e., a person who is 5-foot-10 should weigh between 130 and 175 pounds, and a 6-foot person will range up from that. As an example, let's compare a human body to a house. There's a certain amount of infrastructure—plumbing, heating, electric—that every house needs, and while some have more and some have less, the amount of infrastructure tends to increase proportionately with the size of the house. A taller person requires more mass just to be tall, but that won't translate to an elevated BMI unless the extra weight is disproportionate to the additional height.

BMI Breakdown
<18.5 Underweight
18.5–24.9 Normal
25–29.9 Overweight
30–34.9 Obese
>35 Extremely obese

The beauty of the BMI is that it is simple to measure—all you need is a scale and a measuring tape. The beast of BMI is that although it's a fairly strong predictor of body fatness (particularly at higher BMIs), it leaves out a lot of important body-composition factors, like sex, age, and body type. And though it can suggest that you're carrying extra mass for your height, it can't tell you whether the extra mass is fat or muscle. So the BMI tends to overestimate fat stores for those groups that tend to be leaner: athletes, Black people, men. At the same BMI level, older people tend to have more fat than younger adults, and women tend to have more body fat than men. To that point, the mean body fat percentage for normal-weight women based on BMI (BMI 18–25) is similar to the percentage for men whose BMI is in the obese range (BMI>30).

So if fat is really the problem (and it is), measuring the percentage of body fat is more precise and meaningful than BMI. It can be calculated by a variety of techniques, from large calipers that pinch arm fat, to floating in water, to running a little electricity through your body to see how well you conduct a current. According to the American Council on Exercise, normal body fat for a woman is 25 to 31 percent, and 32 percent or higher is considered obese. For men, the normal body fat is 18 to 24 percent, and 25 percent or more will put you into the hefty class. Note that normal body fat percentage also comes with a range, which tells you that we still don't know exactly what normal is.

The Skinny on the "Obesity Paradox"

If being overweight can shave years off your life, can a person be too skinny? That is the question behind the medical headline–grabbing term "the obesity paradox."

If you graph mortality (the risk of dying) against BMI (body mass index) what you get is a U-shaped curve. That is, people die sooner/younger at low BMIs (Mr. Salty, the pretzel mascot, is too skinny) and at high BMIs (Jabba the Hutt is too fat).

What is mortal about being too skinny? It most likely has to do with the fact that either Mr. Salty has been kept trim by smoking (raising his risk of cardiovascular disease and cancer), or he has been suffering from some other chronic illness that saps his physiology and keeps him from putting more meat on his bones—or salt on his pretzel, as it were. If you are a low-BMI kind of guy who is staying thin by smoking cigarettes, you should quit. That's a bad bargain. On the other hand, if you've been skinny all your life but are otherwise healthy and active, there is no data to suggest that bulking up will do anything to improve your health.

On occasion, controversy arises over what specific BMI or BMI range might be the healthiest. One study made a splash by exposing what it termed "the obesity paradox"—the suggestion that being a little chunky (overweight but not obese) was associated with the lowest mortality. The benefit of having a few calories stored away in case one gets into a metabolic pinch appealed to common sense, but further research put the kibosh on that idea. Across multiple studies, the lowest-mortality BMI seems to be in the 22 to 25 percent range, and it will likely stay that way.

Forgoing the cardiovascular and mortality implications of being overweight, it's simply a lot to carry around. The extra pounds place a heavy toll on joints and can alter our normal body mechanics—the way that our weight and the forces created by our muscles are dispersed through our joints and bones. The archetypal "beer belly" places a lot of strain on the spine, for instance. But because we tend to put on the pounds slowly, this beast of the burden often sneaks up on us. Throw a backpack with 4 gallons of milk on someone who is 32 pounds overweight, and ask them to wear that around 24–7. They will sour on the idea before the milk does.

Location, Location, Location

When it comes to fat, sex matters.

Women have more body fat, and they put it in different places than men. Women preferentially store fat in the skin around their midsection, the physiological basis behind cultural slang such as "thunder thighs" and the complaint that dessert tends to go right to their hips. It's true.

Men, on the other hand, tend to get "Buddha bellies" or "beer bellies": in this case, *some* of the fat is in the skin over the abdomen, but much of it collects inside the abdomen in an area called the "omentum," a thin layer of tissue draping over the intestines. There is a certain mythology that doing sit-ups will get rid of of a beer belly, but other than the calories that are burned off in the process, tightening the abdominal muscles just shoves the omental fat back into the abdomen. Squashing a sleeping bag into a carrier changes its shape but not its mass.

Of note: these sex-based "trendencies" in fat storage are not exclusive contracts: obese men can have thunder thighs, and women can have IPA bellies. Share and share alike.

BMI—and better yet, your percentage of body fat—can tell you how many extra calories you're carrying, but they don't tell you where those calories reside, and location is important. It turns out that a beer belly is much more powerful as a metabolic deranger than large thighs. The diabetic, hypertensive, bad-cholesterol effects that we see with fat seem to come most potently from the omentum, the abdominal fat.

This is why a simple waist measurement can help you understand how risky your weight problem truly is.

Remember, the waist is at level of the iliac crest, the bony prominence that holds your belt up. The hips are what hurt when you lie on your side and try, yet again, to extract the dog's moist and moldy tennis ball from underneath the sofa.

To correctly measure your waist, stand and place a tape measure at belt level around your abdomen. Measure just after you have exhaled. Sucking in is cheating. A waist size greater than 35 inches for women or greater than 40 inches for men portends an increased risk. Yes, some men are slender and some are much more substantial. But beyond early adulthood, the pelvis stops growing, and so any increase in waist size is typically due to expanding omental fat storage.

Turning Green Beans into Blubber

Here it is, the simple key to obesity: when you take in more calories than you spend, your body will store those calories away as fat.

How does a green bean get turned into fat? When it comes to fat, the liver is the CEO of adipose, adipose tissue being the medical term for fat. The liver is capable of converting excess calories *from any food source*—including carbohydrates and protein—into triglycerides, a collection of the three ("tri") fatty acids ("glycerides") that are the primary form of fat storage. Triglycerides can either be stored in the liver or in fat cells in the rest of the body. Again, exactly where that fat is stored on the body has a lot to do with what sex you are and whether you're taking my patented weight-reduction and fat-dissolver pill, Slimminy Glick (call now for a free four-and-a-half-day supply; shipping and handling charges will apply).

Why Do We Eat Too Much?

Well, for most of human history, food was scarce—it was either scattered or not very calorically dense. Try picking wild blueberries. These things are the size of BBs, and the mosquitoes will suck more calories out of you than the berries can give back; no wonder black bears are so ornery. Or sometimes the calories ran away from us when we tried to catch and eat them (damned wooly mammoths!).

This is no longer the issue for many modern humans, particularly in affluent cultures, where food is cheap and lined up neatly on shelves. Like sex, eating food is hardwired into the deepest areas of the brain; and to remind us how important they are, God made both acts pleasurable, a kind of "rewards card" we were handed as a parting gift when we were banished from the Garden of Eden: "Don't forget to eat and procreate!"

We all love to eat—it is a joy, it is a pleasure. So are overeaters actually just weak-minded individuals with no self-discipline or self-control? Probably not. Studies on the hypothalamus—a deep area of the brain that helps us monitor calorie intake and demands and then issues either hunger or satiety ("I'm full") alerts—show that obese people may have a higher so-called "set point" for feeling full. They're not helpless against overeating and they are not Old Country Buffet zombies; but their hunger pangs are more intense, and so for them, weight loss is more difficult. Add to this the fact that modern foods have been specifically formulated to be addictive to optimize sales. The modern food industry's informal assertion "We don't create tastes; we only cater to them" is more than a bit disingenuous (and remarkably similar to pornography industry claims). They know full well that fat, salt, and sugar stimulate reward centers in the brain.

Expanding Convenience, Expanding Waist Lines

The other part of the weight equation—how many calories are spent—is also a modern "success" story. The unstated goal of modernity has been to make life *easier*, which meant that we've ended up burning fewer food calories by burning more coal/oil/gas calories.

The average person spends 25 percent to 30 percent of their daily energy expenditure on muscular activity. But for someone who does physical labor (and that was nearly everyone prior to the Industrial Revolution), that percentage shoots up to 60 or 70 percent. We'll talk more about this in the Move It or Lose It chapter, but the math is simple: burn fewer calories + eat the same = gain weight.

What Should You Weigh?

To review, a scale tells you how much you weigh. The BMI adjusts your weight for your height, which helps, but it still can't tell the difference between fat and muscle. An equation for "Ideal Body Weight" (IBW) uses height but also adjusts for one's sex. Some experts suggest adding 10% to the total if you have a large frame and subtracting 10% for a small frame.

Ideal Body Weight, male:
106 lbs + 6 lbs for every inch over 5 feet

Ideal Body Weight, female:
100 lbs + 5 lbs for every inch over 5 feet

The IBW formula has its drawbacks (including that it underestimates IBW for shorter people, and overestimates IBW for taller people) and it's been largely replaced by the Body Mass Index (BMI). If it's important for you to have a specific weight-loss goal other than the generic "less," you can use the following ideal body weight formula published by a group of researchers in 2016. By plugging in your height and a goal BMI, you can see what your ideal body weight would be for that target BMI. 'If I want to have a BMI of 30, I will need to weigh this much,' etc.

Weight in pounds =
5 x BMI + [BMI/5 x (height in inches -- 60)]

In any case, this isn't Olympic boxing, where you need to make a certain weight or you're out. You're trying to get to a reasonable, healthy weight. That raises the question, "What's the best way to get there?"

"Diet" Is a Four-Letter Word: And Also a Transitive Verb

Like tabloid marriages, crazy weight loss stories make for interesting press, but they rarely hold up long term. You're not going on a diet, you're trying to change the way you eat and exercise forever—or the lost weight will surely return. The word "diet" is a transitory verb, as in "I went on a vacation in Mexico." But then your vacation ended and you came home to the harried, frantic life you've always led. Vacation over. Nothing really changed. You went on a diet and then you came back. And nothing really changed.

But if you are going to lose weight permanently, you'll need to make permanent changes, i.e., ones that are sustainable. Witness the classic New Year's resolution to "hit the gym" that leaves you so sore by the third week of January that you're grinding up ibuprofen pills and pounding them out into tortillas. They taste better that way and slide down easier, especially with meat, sour cream, and salsa.

A Buffet of Diet Options

There are so many diet plans out there that it can be difficult to keep them all straight. But the nuts and bolts of all of them tend to revolve around the same three major caloric sources:

- Carbohydrates (starches and sugars)
- Protein (meats, beans, and nuts)
- Fat (both amount and type—saturated or unsaturated)

Here's a brief rundown on the most common diet options.

Low-Fat Diet

This is the easy one, and perhaps the oldest. As I mentioned in the chapter on nutrition, when our collective arteries started clogging up with atherosclerosis, we assumed that dietary fat was the issue. And because fat has the highest concentration of calories, it made sense that fat was making us fat. One truism in nutrition is: when we stop eating from one particular food group, we don't stop eating; we just eat more items from the other food groups. When we ditched fat, we pivoted to eating more carbohydrates, often highly refined carbs that turn out to behave more like metabolic gunpowder. Avoiding fats of all kinds (even healthy plant oils) in favor of carbohydrates left us fatter—and more unhealthy—than ever.

Diabetic Diet

Like the low-fat diet, this one has been around a while. Because diabetics have high blood sugar, the diabetic diet avoids sugars. Growing up, I remember seeing an explosion of food products that were endorsed by the American Diabetes Association. It seemed like diabetics needed to be eating a lot of special foods. But as food research has improved, a "diabetic diet" closely approximates what we should all be eating: fruits and vegetables, proteins that are light on saturated fat, and complex (high-glycemic-index) carbohydrates rather than highly processed (low-glycemic-index) carbohydrates, the pinnacle of which is plain old everyday sugar.

Low-Carb Diet (paleo, high-protein, ketogenic/Atkins diet)

The idea that one could lose weight chomping down on steak, bacon, and butter makes this diet very attractive to men and carnivores. How could a diet that increases saturated fat intake really work? It turns out that the deleterious effects of extra fat intake are more than offset by the healthy benefits of weight loss. And the diet made famous by Robert Atkins has one unique claim to fame: it's the only diet plan in which weight loss isn't accompanied by hunger pangs. One of the critical jobs of the liver is to provide the body with a steady supply of glucose. It typically does this by burning up carbs, which (as noted previously) are essentially chains of sugars. If carb sources are low, or a person is fasting, the liver breaks down fat to produce an alternative fuel called "ketones." Research consistently shows that these ketones suppress the secretion of the hunger hormone ghrelin and increase the release of satiety ("I'm full") peptides. This happens even when you're taking exogenous ketones—that is, ketones in a pill form (there are many of these out there).

A word on the paleo diet. This gets grouped in with other low-carb diets, but it is slightly different. As the name suggests, the paleo diet tries to recreate what humans were eating during the Paleolithic era, back when we were hunter-gatherers, and before we were farmers. So the paleo diet leaves out major carbohydrate sources like grains (wheat, oats, barley), legumes (beans, lentils, peanuts and peas), and sugar; and it doesn't include dairy products because the Holsteins of the Paleolithic era certainly weren't going to let you milk them. This leaves the paleo plate piled high with forager fare: fruits, vegetables, nuts and seeds, lean meats, and fish—a pretty healthy platter.

Intermittent fasting

This might be better labeled as the "Would-you-please-quit-eating-all-the-time?! Diet," although it's not your typical diet plan. It's more about *how often* one eats rather than *what* one eats.

Intermittent fasting does share certain philosophical features with the paleo diet in that it mimics how our ancestors ate—intermittently, as food sources became available, since there were no cupboards, fridges, or freezers. It shares metabolic features with low carb/high protein diets, as both approaches push our bodies to burn fats and ketones for fuel. In our current, 3-meals-a-day-plus-nibblies culture, just about the time we've burned through all the sugar supplies from our last meal and are beginning to burn some of our Strategic Fat Reserves, we start eating again. D'oh!

'Fasting' is a fancy word for not eating, and our forebearers (even relatively recently) spent a lot of time not eating. They were good at it, and a bevy of research in both animals and humans shows that fasting is good for us. Switching to this fat-burning metabolism seems to have a host of health benefits, as it improves glucose regulation, increases resistance to stress, and suppresses inflammation. It appears to be the antithesis of the metabolic syndrome described earlier in this chapter.

One approach to intermittent fasting is to establish a daily time slot for eating—perhaps a 10-hour period to start, tapering to a daily 6-hour period a few months down the line. Another approach is called "5:2," where one eats normally for five days a week, and sharply reduces caloric intake on the other two days.

When first initiating an intermittent fast regimen, most people will experience hunger, irritability, and problems concentrating during their fasts, but that usually resolves in a month. As a weight loss method, intermittent fasting doesn't seem superior to any other weight loss plans.

If starvation is not eating enough, and nowadays most of us are eating too much, then perhaps intermittent fasting—the widely spaced dinner bell of the ancients—can bring us to healthier ground.

Mediterranean Diet

Researchers first studied dietary habits in Italy and Greece because of the natives' lower incidence of cardiovascular disease. What kept them there was the food—a tasty mix of vegetables, whole grains (complex carbohydrates!), fruits, beans, nuts and seeds, fish, and olive oil (a healthy, monounsaturated oil). What they don't eat is a lot of red meat or dairy products. It can be difficult to tease out the health benefits of a particular culture's diet from other health-promoting activities in that culture. For one, what are the benefits of living in a place where a sunny, temperate climate boosts the mood and allows for regular physical activity in a culture that was designed for foot traffic rather than the automobile? Happily, the Mediterranean diet's health benefits have held up very well when exported to harsher climes. It may well be the way we were designed to eat. Geologists have not yet found potato chips anywhere in the fossil record.

Please Pass the Myths; I'd Like to Try One

It's hard to know whether there is more mythology surrounding the Kennedy family or the weight-loss industry, but in early 2013, an NIH-sponsored study examined some of the most common myths behind obesity and weight loss. I've quoted (or, in some cases, paraphrased) the most interesting ones and then added comments.

Myth #1
Small changes in calorie intake or exercise will produce consistent long-term weight loss.

Not true: the human body adapts to a new calorie-scarce environment by becoming more metabolically efficient, which means the pounds come off harder over time. This is called "diet-induced adaptive thermogenesis." Seasoned dieters call it "my personal experience." The study specifically debunks the commonly touted rule of thumb that a 500-calorie deficit each day will lead to a one-pound weight loss each week. Maybe in the short term, but probably not in the long term.

Myth #2
Modest weight-loss goals work better.

Nope. At least there is nothing in the scientific literature to support that. Individuals approach weight loss differently, but go ahead, dream big—or rather, dream small, as in smaller waist size.

Myth #3
Slow and steady weight loss (the turtle) beats fast and big weight loss (the hare).

Also nope. There are a lot of ways to the finish line, and this is not a timed event. Fast or slow can work.

Myth #4
Don't start a weight-loss program until you're ready.

Nah. Start as soon as you can—you may never be ready.

Myth #5
Physical Education class keeps kids from getting fat.

Nice theory, but it isn't working—certainly not at the current allotted time or intensity of PE class.

Myth #6
Breastfeeding lowers a child's risk of becoming an obese adult.

Slurping up the vanilla nipple ripple has a host of health benefits, but weight control is not one of them. If you're still blaming your weight problems on being fed formula as an infant, give it up.

Myth #7
Sex is a good way to burn 100 to 300 calories.

It is if you have to walk someplace to get it. Nice try! There are a lot of variables in play, but the act burns 21 kcal for a 30-something male under average conditions.

The study then went on to list a series of unproven presumptions, like the idea that recurrent weight loss and weight gain (so-called "yo-yoing") leads to higher mortality, or that skipping breakfast is the key, or that snacking leads to weight gain. Before you give up and slit your wrists with the sharpened end of a French fry carton, the review finishes with some encouraging weight-loss information.

Heritage is not destiny: You might come from a super-sized family, but you're not predestined to live like one.

Diets work in the short term, but fail in the long term. Don't diet. Change the way you eat.

Move it to lose it: Exercise, in sufficient quantities, does aid in weight loss (and improves health even if it doesn't lead to actual weight loss).

Food focus: Structured, nutritious meals lead to better weight loss. This is probably the appeal of weight-loss programs that provide meals. Focus on the quality of food, not just the quantity. Cheap prepared foods tend to be unhealthy.

Diet drugs are like toupees: They work as long as you continue to use them.

There are four FDA-approved prescription medications for weight loss, but they are not widely used due to cost and side effects. And like all quick fixes, the weight comes back if and when people stop using them.

...if you go on a diet, there's the very notion of going, "Well then, one day I will come off this diet." And it's not about that. I mean, I have done every diet under the sun. I've done them all. I've done shake-in-the-morning, shake-in-the-evening, cabbage soup. They work in the short term, and then, if anything, I've always put on more weight after that."
—*James Corden on CBS Mornings*

MOVE IT (YOUR BODY) OR LOSE IT (YOUR GOOD HEALTH)

The Perils of a Sitty Disposition, and the Need to Exorcise Your Inner Slacker Demons. Keep Moving!

I haven't been in a gym or fitness center since medical school, but as an English major and word nerd, I like to mentally collect the kind of motivational signs that end up on the walls of workout rooms: No Pain, No Gain; Tough Times Don't Last, Tough People Do; or Pain Is Temporary, Pride Is Forever. Are you there to get in shape, or suffer?

You don't see really honest signs like, Admit it: You're Here Because You Feel Fat and Sleepy, or Your Body Is a Temple, but the Temple Is in Need of Major Renovations, or If You're Trying to Outrun the Grim Reaper, You've Already Been Lapped.

The one workout sign that still seems like good advice is Move It, or Lose It. In a remarkable way, this describes the plight of the modern, affluent human: cloaked in convenience, killed by comfort. Exertion of any kind has been typecast as arduous and painful, and so when humanity came face-to-face with the mountain of effort it took to get our lazy asses off the couch to change

MAN OVERBOARD!

Sitting is unhealthy. NEAT (non-exercise activity thermogenesis) is the physical activity you pass up every day in favor of convenience. It's the low-hanging activity fruit, so pick it! Stand. Walk. Climb stairs. And when does "being active" become "exercise"?

the TV channel, the gods mercifully intervened and the television remote was born. And the electric can opener, because it's just too much effort to open a can by hand.

Serial advancements in the twentieth century—the dawn of convenience—were topped off by the Computer-Internet Revolution, which brought nearly everything we needed into our laps and laptops. We don't even have to get up to answer the phone anymore.

Does scrubbing grease [off a frying pan] feel like a workout? Scrub less with Dawn Ultra.
—*TV commercial*

If scrubbing a pan feels like a workout, you definitely need more workouts and less Dawn Ultra. When the day comes when we can poop or pee into our computer, and food can be downloaded through a USB port, the paralysis will be complete. Homo sapiens, the goofy-looking, hairless ape creature that used its superior brain and rather modest physical capabilities—sturdy legs and a pair of opposable thumbs—to populate the world, will be functionally reduced to a brain encased in blubber. Was the movie *Wall-E* a dystopian satire, prophetic voice, or both?

The problem is, that superior brain of ours requires the rest of the body to support it, and there's more and more evidence that the modern human body runs best under the conditions set out in the owner's manual for the original human body: stay lean, keep physically active, subsist on a natural diet of simple foods, and maintain strong communal ties. These are the traits of people living in so-called "Blue Zones," five specific geographic pockets in the world where people live long *and well.* Many of the rest of us are living overweight, underactive, socially estranged lives, as we nibble on foods that have been pistol-whipped by food chemist vigilantes. Two cornerstones of the human success story—the ability to do physical work, and the ability to capture calories—have been radically undermined by today's endless convenience and limitless access to calories.

NEAT: Non-Exercise Activity Thermogenesis

When I hear the claim, "I eat the same things he does, and *he* doesn't get fat," I generally conclude that the person who is making this disclaimer doesn't really understand what he is eating. This view is bolstered by patients I see in the hospital who are struggling with profound obesity and its aftermath, and who claim to be subsisting on rice cakes and Diet Coke.

They're not lying; they're just not keeping track, or they are ashamed of how much they really do eat. Either way, their claims cannot possibly be true, for the following reasons.

About 60 percent of our daily energy expenditure goes to basic housekeeping, that is, into keeping all of our organs powered up and running. We call this the "basal metabolic rate." As with heating a home, the larger a person is, the larger the heating bills. The larger the body, the more energy it takes just to maintain that body, and that body weight. So you can't nibble your way up to 400 pounds and then keep it there without shoveling a lot of coal into the furnace. The math doesn't work. A *sedentary* 50-year-old, six-foot male weighing 300 pounds would need to eat 3300 kcal per day just to maintain that weight; if he decided to get a little more active, let's say for less than 1 hour per day, he'd need 3700 kcal just to keep from losing weight.

About 10 percent of our daily energy needs go to digesting food: splicing and dicing it, mixing and absorbing it, and then distributing it to different organs throughout the body. This doesn't vary much person to person. For a completely sedentary, inert person, this 60 percent to keep the lights on and 10 percent to digest food would be the entire daily energy bill.

An average person (average weight, average activity level) burns about 3,000 kcals every day, so about 2,100 kcal (or 70 percent) is for basic metabolism and food digestion, and 900 kcal is spent on physical activity. Surprisingly, a small portion of that—around 100 kcal— is spent on what one might call purposeful exercise: going for a run, working out. The remaining 800 kcal is what Dr. James Levine, for 20 years a world-renowned leader in obesity research at Mayo Clinic, calls "non-exercise activity thermogenesis," or NEAT.

To clarify this "I don't eat what you eat so how come I'm still heavier than you?" quandary, Levine conducted two very sophisticated studies that he details in his book, *Move a Little, Lose a Lot.*

In the first study, Levine and his colleagues spent 8 weeks giving fifteen volunteers (and also himself) an extra 1,000 calories, each and every day. That's the equivalent of a Big Mac and a large shake. The researchers used highly sophisticated techniques to keep track of the volunteers' caloric expenditures, even measuring the calories in volunteers' stool to see if some people were, quite literally, dumping calories. (That's not a ridiculous notion: it's increasingly clear that the bacteria in our colon play a role in how thick or thin we are).

By the end of the study, one volunteer gained barely an ounce, one gained 14 pounds, and the others fell somewhere in between. Why were some storing away those extra calories and others burning them? The answer was NEAT: some volunteers stayed more active than others.

To answer that question in more detail, Levine did a second study where he outfitted 10 lean volunteers and 10 mildly obese volunteers with what he termed "NEAT underwear," technology that measured volunteers' every movement, every half-second, for 10 days. Volunteers were instructed to stick to their usual routine, and to not attend any sit-ins or go on an exercise rager. You can guess the punchline: the mildly obese volunteers were more sedentary, spending an average of 2.5 hours a day longer in the seated or reclined position than lean volunteers—a difference of about 350 calories a day (the equivalent of 60 minutes of aerobics, or a 45-minute run).

Stand Up. Keep It Moving!

Simply put, those who stayed lean kept moving, and the idea of *keep moving* is what encompasses Levine's NEAT philosophy. His message is a blast from the past: to be who we are engineered to be, we must reclaim some key aspects of the agrarian life that we surrendered to the computer age. To illustrate, an average Old Order Amish male

MAN OVERBOARD!

takes 18,000 steps each day (about 9 miles) and his wife takes about 14,000 (7 miles). For comparison, the average desk-bound American takes about 5,000 to 6,000 steps in a day.

Levine's recipe for health and happiness is a hopeful, relatively simple, and eminently achievable one: reclaim the simple activities that we were born to do. Stand up. Keep moving.

The idea is not to develop a neurotic, pacing-the-cage mentality in which sitting down to watch a movie fills one with anxiety and self-loathing. What Levine champions is that there is time for NEAT if you simply do the things you need to do while getting the activity that you need or want.

You can walk at a very leisurely pace, 1 mph even, and watch your favorite TV show. You can surf the Internet while stepping up on your old StairMaster. With cellphones, you can answer all your phone calls on the go. Have walking meetings. Do your computer work standing up. Take the stairs rather than the elevator. Scrub a greasy pan. Drive by the drive-thru: get out of the car to pick up your prescription.

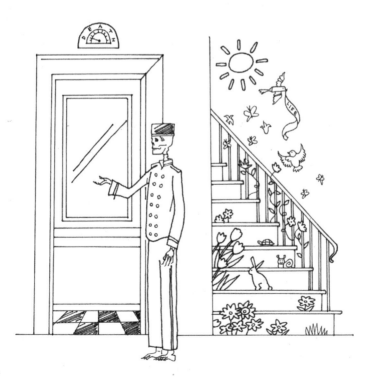

Don't eat at your desk. Walk to a destination and then eat. Rather than letting the dog out in the backyard, take her for a walk. If you want to get healthy or stay healthy, you need to be active, and NEAT is the low-hanging fruit.

For a culture bursting at the seams, or buying ever larger seams so they don't burst, the take-home message from Levine's experiment is that weight gain is really an imbalance between diet (energy intake) and activity (energy use). In the current paradigm, we tend to make food the villain: there's way too much of it, and it tastes too good. We are far less likely to blame the extra pounds on Dawn Ultra, an elevator, our car, the drive-up window, the electric can opener, the golf cart we use to grab the mail. In our recent evolution, we have de-evolved, but we can change that.

Staying Active Sheds Pounds, but Is There More to It Than That?

Data collected by devices in the U.S. National Health and Nutrition Examination Survey (NHANES) indicate that children and adults spend approximately 7.7 hours per day (55 percent of their monitored waking time) being sedentary.

It's easy to find good scientific data on what the sedentary life does to us. Simply go to the studies that were designed to measure the benefits of exercise and look at the control group, the participants who didn't do anything but just sit around.

A 2011 review out of Duke University did exactly that and found that the participants randomized to the sedentary group metabolically deteriorated during the study period. The key driver of their physiologic demise was weight or fat gain, and they put it on in the worst place, in the belly. The extra fat brought with it a whole bunch of metabolic problems, such as higher glucose, higher insulin levels, and more LDL—the "bad cholesterol."

Since a third of the US population is overweight, and a third is obese, the principal perceived benefit of exercise is to lose weight. But physical activity has many benefits that are independent of its weight loss effects, including lower rates of heart disease, strokes, and some cancers. It improves joint, bone and muscle health, even in the presence of disease (arthritis, for example). Movement also seems to be really good for the brain. Physical activity causes an increase in blood flow to the brain; it reduces depression and slows cognitive decline in older folks.

In offices where Levine has done NEAT makeovers, employees become more productive (which of course is the true measure of any employee). This symbiotic mind-body connection is why Levine states in *Move a Little, Lose a Lot*, "Mental health, I believe, is the most profound argument for NEAT." In 2020, the US Department of Health and Human Services updated its 2008 Physical Activity Guidelines to include new scientific evidence proving that physical activity is Popeye's spinach for the human brain, not just for muscles. Physical activity improves cognition (thinking), depression, anxiety, sleep and overall quality of life.

If better brain health doesn't get your attention, how about premature death? Let me put you inside a graph from the 2020 Physical Activity Guidelines.

You're standing at home plate in a baseball field where the left field corner is a deep red color—the highly mortal Gorge of Eternal Peril. The right field corner is the healthy deep green of lower mortality semi-eternal life.

Sitting too much pulls you off home plate and into the rising, orange-red mortality of third base. Sitting *all* the time will land you in the high-mortality left-field corner, and from there it will take lots of moderate-to-vigorous physical activity to overcome your "sitty" disposition and slide you into the nearest green out in center field. On the other hand, if you stay active and don't sit around too much, just modest amounts of physical activity will get you off home plate and put you in life-affirming green before you even get to first base.

To put it another way, what's more life-threatening, lots of sitting or no exercise? Sitting is! A NEAT life doesn't preclude exercising, but if exercising isn't for you, at least keep moving!

Telomere Talk

As sophisticated as modern medicine has become, we can only tell people's chronological (calendar) age, not their true, physiologic/biologic age. We can count out candles on a cake, but that doesn't measure how fast or slow we are aging at the tissue level.

Now researchers have the ability to measure telomeres, which are sections of DNA that cap each end of our chromosomes (the strands that carry the genetic blueprint for each cell). Telomeres get shorter as we age. "Like sands through the hourglass… so are the days of our lives." Telomeres act as a biological clock for each cell.

There is now an intriguing body of evidence showing that, like a spendy hair-conditioning product, staying active seems to keep telomeres longer and full of body. In an article in the *Archives of Internal Medicine,* researchers studied more than 2,400 pairs of white British twins, most of them women, and asked them to fill out questionnaires detailing their physical activity level during their work and leisure time over the previous 12 months. Participants also completed a questionnaire designed to assess current and retrospective physical activity in their twenties.

Researchers measured telomere lengths in participants' white blood cells and found a strongly positive association between the level of activity during leisure time and the length of the telomeres. In other words, "Move it, or lose telomere length." In fact, the most active subjects (who engaged in three hours of moderate to vigorous activity per week) had the same average telomere length as sedentary individuals (who exercised for 16 minutes or less per week) who were as much as 10 years younger.

Acknowledging that telomere length and longevity might have a strong genetic component, the researchers looked at a subset of 67 pairs of twins who were raised together but were living different lifestyles in terms of physical activity. They found similar results—that is, the twin who exercised more had longer telomeres than the more sedentary twin.

The researchers drew their conclusions based on reporting of physical activity in leisure time. Surprisingly, the amount of physical activity at work didn't seem to have an effect on telomere length. That might have something to do with the well-demonstrated telomere-chomping effect of stress, and just might add validity to the oft-heard claim, "This job is killing me!" Learning this, Levine comes in and provides everyone a treadmill desk (not a treadmill test), which allows workers to stand up and walk while doing their office work.

When Does Being "Active" Transition to Exercise?

As I will discuss in the Rise Up, AARPathletes! chapter, activity is good, but exercise is better. When does one become the other? Because I consider light-intensity activities to be nearly effortless, and because activity recommendations from the bigwigs all start with moderate-intensity activities, that's where I think activity becomes exercise.

Here is a summary of the four levels of activity, with individual clues to recognize which one you're in.

Not Active

This activity level is characterized by a pervasive non-activity, and is often described as a state of physical inertness that feels effortless—because it is. Can be achieved in a seated or reclined position; or while floating in the pool on your partner's inflatable chaise lounge.

Sense of exertion scale: 0 (zero)

Metabolic equivalent of task (MET) level (a measure of energy expenditure for any activity): 1

Heart rate ("pulse"): in the resting range, 60–100.

Active (Light-Intensity Activity)

These include many of the non-strenuous daily activities that are the mainstay of a NEAT approach to life. Walking at a leisurely 2 mph is a common example. It's the kind of walk where you can stare off into the distance, let your mind wander, critique the neighbors' landscaping and appalling lack of taste.

Sense of exertion scale: 1–4 (out of 10)

MET level: 1–3.0

Percentage of maximum heart rate (which is calculated as 220 − your age): 45— 63 percent

Moderate Exercise (Moderate-Intensity Activities)

Walking 3 mph means you are now exercising. You are reaching a level of physical activity that requires conscious effort, where you need to deliberately push to maintain your pace. At this level of exercise, one can talk but not sing.

Sense of exertion scale: 5–6

MET level: 3.0–5.9

Percentage of maximum heart rate: 64-76 percent

Vigorous Exercise (Vigorous-Intensity Activity)

Running a mile in 10 minutes (6 mph) will get you to this peak level. The oxygen or breathing demands at this level mean you still can't sing, and you probably can't say more than a few words at a time.

Sense of exertion scale: 7–10

MET level: 10 or higher

Percentage of maximum heart rate: 77-93 percent

Do What You Can, as Much as You Can. Do What Fits You.

Do the moderate and vigorous levels of exercise seem intimidating, unobtainable, or more than that, just plain uninteresting?

If so, I'll spend the next chapter, Rise Up, AARPathletes!, trying to convince you that breaking a sweat and getting winded every once in a while might be a healthy idea that's entirely within your grasp. If I fail, you can rest—or preferably, stand—assured that by avoiding excessive sitting time and becoming a "NEAT freak," you'll reap the health benefits of being active while keeping your telomeres as long and as lush as possible.

In the end, we all have to figure it out for ourselves, and the pom-poms that matter most are the ones we wave on our own behalf.

12 RISE UP, AARPATHLETES!
Activity Is Good; Exercise Is Better

If you're a committed "non-athlete" and fixin' to skip this chapter, please read this first.

Okay, you don't consider yourself an exerciser. It's just not you. You hate running. You don't have the social temperament or the body image to show up in a gym. You're not interested in doing a Turkey Trot, Reindeer Run or, God forbid, the Boston Marathon. You'd almost certainly drown in a triathlon. You just want to walk your one or two miles a day, or ride your stationary bike and leave it at that.

Fine. I get it. You're on board with trying to live an active, NEAT-freak life, but you don't see yourself becoming an AAR-Pathlete ("ar-PATH-leet"), or any kind of athlete. Let me explain why I think you should at least *consider* adding a little huffing and pufffing to your life.

●●●●●●●●●●●●

I'm no sadist, but I do get an embarrassing sense of satisfaction when a young but aging professional athlete gets injured during a routine, seemingly innocuous play.

At age 38, Yankees franchise shortstop

MAN OVERBOARD!

Aging is a perpetual challenge for the AARPathlete. But go for the bronze! You're not fragile; you're inactive. You can't grow hair, but you can grow muscle! Tackle the Fab Four: aerobic fitness, resistance training, flexibility, and balance. Intensity of training is more important than duration. Mortality benefit of exercise eventually levels off, but health benefits continue.

Derek Jeter broke his ankle fielding a ground ball. At 42, Mariano Rivera—perhaps the greatest relief pitcher in the history of baseball—tore his ACL shagging fly balls in batting practice. At 35, the now legendary Kobe Bryant—the blueprint for a professional athlete—ruptured his Achilles tendon during a routine drive to his left. Later that year, he fractured his left knee (tibia) in a game against the Memphis Grizzlies.

If these extraordinarily gifted athletes can get old, then it can surely happen to you and me. It *will* happen to you and me. It *is* happening to you and me.

Whatever kind of athlete you are, or were, the human athletic performance trajectory hits a peak around age 30 to 35 (depending on the person and the sport), and then begins a downward slide starting in the forties.

The decline is not a black diamond slope with moguls. It starts out like a green beginner trail, which provides some time for quietly schussing through the powdery back bowls of denial. But the decline becomes more blue intermediate as one enters the pre-geezer years. The lesson here is: enjoy the view from the top of the mountain for as long as you have it. Today is as young as you'll ever be.

In the movie *The Princess Bride*, it's Count Rugen's crudely demonic, suction cup torture machine that literally sucks the years out of our hero Westley, whose favorite sport is swashbuckling. The physiology of aging is considerably more complicated than the Count's device, which was powered by a Flintstones-era water wheel. The natural aging process can be more gentle and doesn't generally involve agonizing pain. Although we age on a cellular level and across all of our tissues simultaneously, what we most often feel is the loss of muscle power (strength and quickness) and cardiovascular fitness (energy and endurance). The two are intimately linked, but let's look at them individually.

Aging Muscles and Motor Units

A muscle group—the biceps muscle for instance—is a collection of thousands and sometimes hundreds of thousands of muscle fibers. (Genetics determine how many fibers a person has in a muscle group, and how "muscular" any individual might be.) The length of these fibers increases until we reach adulthood, and after that, these fibers can either wither ("atrophy") or bulk up ("hypertrophy"), depending on how often and how hard they are used. The size of the fiber isn't everything: speed and force of contraction is important too.

Groups of muscle fibers are stimulated by "motor units," tiny nerves that die out over time, leaving the muscle fibers they serve without any neurological stimulation. Without the stimulus to fire and contract, the muscle fibers also die off. Undoubtedly, aging muscle deteriorates for other reasons too—decreased hormonal stimulation from testosterone and growth hormone, or intrinsic muscle-aging changes—but the loss of neural stimulation seems to play a major role.

There are three main types of muscle fibers, which some PhD genius creatively labeled Type I, Type IIa and Type IIb.

- Type I is a slow-twitch fiber, better suited for endurance
- Type IIa is a fast-twitch fiber that runs on oxygen ("aerobic")
- Type IIb is a fast-twitch fiber that doesn't require oxygen ("anaerobic")

The die-off of motor units seems to primarily involve those going to the fast and powerful Type II muscle fibers, rather than the slow-but-steady Type I fibers. The subsequent loss of strength and power is a real kick in the shorts to many athletic endeavors, with the notable exceptions of billiards, shuffleboard, and cribbage. That also explains why, for example, "clean and jerk" weight lifting performance drops off sooner than marathon performance.

Our muscle strength peaks around age 30, and begins to decline at age 50. For sedentary couch surfers, muscle strength declines roughly 15 percent per decade between the ages of 50 and 70, and 30 percent per decade after that.

Sucking Air: VO2 Max

One of the touching Hallmark moments of aging is finding yourself sucking air after something as innocuous as walking *all the way* up from the basement to the second floor. Didn't use to do that. Never noticed that before. Did I slip on ankle weights rather than socks this morning?

That shortness of breath you're feeling is a craving for oxygen. It's weird to consider, but our bodies are doing a slow burn. Like a crackling fire, we use oxygen to burn fuel—which in our case is the food we eat, not firewood. As mentioned before, we do have some muscle fibers that burn certain fuels without oxygen ("anaerobic metabolism"). They are good for short bursts of speed and strength, but they quickly fatigue. Most muscle fibers—and virtually all other tissue in our body— rely on oxygen-based, "aerobic metabolism," which is why exercising makes us breathe harder.

Although getting winded might seem like a lung thing, it's your body demanding more oxygen, and the oxygen delivery system involves more than your lungs. If you have workout buddies who are on the more serious side of things, or just techy, or just ridiculously analytical (where a workout is a 45-minute stare-down with their Apple Watch), you may have heard the term "VO2 max." This refers to the maximum amount of oxygen that your body can pluck from the air, deliver to the body, and burn. There are multiple factors involved in what your VO2 max might be—lung function, and how good your muscles are at extracting oxygen and glucose off the conveyor belt of your bloodstream are two of them—but the key factor is the strength of one's heart, the giant pump that is picking up oxygenated blood from the lungs and distributing it to the entire body. That's why VO2 max is said to be the most specific measurement of one's cardiovascular ("cardio") fitness—that is, of one's athletic, aerobic fitness.

Not that you're considering it, but here's how "blood doping" works: if you've trained as hard as you can, to the point where your heart can't pump any harder than it already is, then one way to increase oxygen delivery is to increase your red blood cells (the primary carriers of oxygen in the bloodstream). You can do that by getting a transfusion, but if you get caught, you might have to give up your Tour de France jackets and Sheryl Crow.

The sad news is that VO2 max declines at a rate of 5 percent to 15 percent per decade after the age of 25. The good news is that endurance training can mitigate that decline, and increase maximal oxygen consumption by 10 percent to 30 percent in some individuals.

Golf as a "Sport" and the Subtleties of Aging

A decline in cardiovascular fitness and muscle power are major factors in the decline of the aging AARPathlete, which is why exercise recommendations—like those from the American College of Sports Medicine (ACSM)—always include aerobic exercise (three to five days per week for 20 to 60 minutes) and resistance (muscle) training (two to three days per week).

But the physical decline we experience with aging plays out in a myriad of other ways, which is why the ACSM also recommends both flexibility and balance training two to three days per week. These more subtle areas of decline are neatly illustrated by the "sport" of golf.

Professional golfers are not immune to injury, but until the PGA makes golf a contact sport, or adds a time component that requires golfers to sprint through the entire course, most of their injuries will remain relatively minor and related to repetitive motion or overuse, or by something that happened far off the course. Tiger Woods seriously injured his back when he got tired of being Tiger Woods and started training with the Navy Seals.

So in a high-finesse, but rigorously non-rigorous "sport" like golf, where mental things like concentration, shot and club selection, and swing adjustment are so key, why does the Senior Tour start at age 50? Because aging diminishes our reflexes, coordination, balance, depth perception, flexibility, and the elastic recoil of tendons and ligaments. The golfers in the Senior Tour are hardly nursing home material, and their accumulated wisdom of the game is worth a few strokes, but the athletic precision required by their profession amplifies the tiny physiologic and anatomic deductions that time applies to each of us. Senior golfers have holes or even rounds where they could keep pace with their younger selves, but as with 50-year-old Phil Mickelson's victory in the 2021 PGA Championship, these are the exceptions, not the rule.

This is why the American College of Sports Medicine includes flexibility and balance in its exercise regimen. Flexibility isn't just for contortionists or ballet dancers. It helps keep our tendons (binding muscle to bone) and ligaments (binding bone to bone) healthier. It helps keep our bodies in ergonomic balance. If you think about it, every muscle or muscle group has a partner that it must work with, and not against. When you lean over to tie your shoes, your abdominal muscles must contract, but the muscles along the back of the spine must also relax. It's the reverse when you stand up. When you flex your bicep, the tricep must relax.

If you are still in the active denial phase of your maturing life, here are a host of very logical, *very* plausible, *even believable* explanations for why someone with your renowned physical gifts may be starting to suck.

A Partial Litany of Reasons I'm Starting to Suck Athletically

- Job stress
- "The kids/adult children are sucking the life out of me." (KACSLOOM)
- Sleep deprivation, due to KACSLOOM, and also job
- Have not updated athletic equipment since college
- Genetic factors, including sloth and nihilism
- Subtle fluctuations in the short term bond market
- Chafing
- Gluten. *Damn you, gluten*
- Gluten-free foods
- Climate change
- Hops leaching away critical but yet-to-be-discovered micronutrients.

This list is by no means complete, but having a list of poor performance excuses memorized and at the ready can be handy when you're getting your ass handed to you by the local peloton; or when you're running a 10k and it seems like the pavement beneath your feet is—no kidding, this has happened to me!—*sliding forward*, which, as frustrating as that may be, is at least an explanation for why you're working so hard to run that slow.

　　　　　　　　　　　　　　　　　　　　　　MAN OVERBOARD!

Sticking the Landing. What'll It Be: The Fountain at Caesar's Palace, or 13 Buses at Wembley Stadium?

Alright, so the decline in muscle function and cardiovascular fitness looks like the exit ramp on a stunt jump by your childhood hero Evel Knievel, who, incidentally, died at age 69 of diabetes, liver disease, pulmonary fibrosis, and what pathologists termed "general abuse."

The good news is that each of us has some say in the matter of this "controlled" crash landing into the everlasting. We hold some sway over whether we land short, like Evel at Caesar's Palace, where we tumble over the handlebars and break a bunch of bones and spend a month in a publicity-induced coma, or whether we clear 13 buses at London's Wembley Stadium but *still* end up crashing and breaking a pelvis—although not badly enough to keep us from walking back up the ramp, with assistance, to the raucous cheers of the crowd.

But hey, Knievel landed most of his jumps, and so can you. There *will* be a decline, an off-ramp, but there doesn't have to be a crash. You do get some say over where you land on the infamous "All-Cause Mortality" (i.e., death for any reason) curve, so keep these points in mind:

- For the inert/sedentary individuals, low levels of activity bring the biggest gains (i.e. mortality drops most sharply with small improvements in activity).
- Being active and exercising drops the risk of dying *early* by 30 percent to 40 percent. (And just to be clear, the risk of dying in this life is 100 percent, a certainty, although scientists are working on changing that.)
- Yes, the mortality benefits of exercise stall out—i.e., you can't exercise yourself to Eternal Life—but there's more to life than how old you are when you die (quantity): there's how well you lived (quality) and exercise can increase that.

It seems too good to be true, but it is: physical activity improves just about every single health outcome that we can name. Note that some of those benefits arrive in the long term, some in the short. Squeezing in a workout when there didn't seem to be time for it won't do much to lower your long-term cancer risk, but it will reduce the stress of that day, and help you sleep better that night. Here are a couple of other benefits that didn't make the list.

Exercise helps build physical reserves. The more you have, the more you can afford to lose. Having some physical reserves will help you better weather an illness, injury, or some other life event that landed you in the penalty box.

Having a little something extra in the fitness bag can help you avoid injury. The aging body can do a lot, but it doesn't like surprises. It likes consistency. Over-exertion invites injury, and over-exertion happens more easily if you're not in shape.

Staying fit can make it safer and easier to say "yes" to spontaneous things. Like a pick-up basketball game, a soccer game at a picnic, or something "non-athletic," like helping the neighbor with some heavy lifting on a deck project. Staying in shape can make it easier to train up to something special, like hiking a "14'er" with friends, doing a mini-triathlon with a college buddy, or signing up for a weekend-long bike ride fundraiser.

It's critically important to remember that although the mortality benefits of exercise fade out at a certain level, the health benefits do not. Exercise offers the option of a healthier life, just not eternal life.

"The [health] benefits continue to increase when a person does more than the equivalent of 300 minutes a week of moderate-intensity aerobic activity. Research has not identified an upper limit of total activity, above which additional health benefits cease to occur."

Your aging body is making you an offer you cannot refuse, but you do have some choices. You can fight the decline, and if you've been inactive for a series of decades, you can recover some of what you've lost. VO2 max can be improved. Yes, it's true that older, geezer muscle is less responsive to resistance exercise training, but it is not unresponsive to exercise. Researchers put a small group of men in their early 70's on a 12-week resistance training program. Leg strength improved 25-30% and muscle biopsies showed that Type 2 muscle fibers—the fast ones that give us power—had increased in size, while the slow-twitch Type 1 fibers remained the same.

Nowadays, Most Work Is Not Exercise

My father labored hard as a "facility operations" guy and he liked active work. But I cannot conjure up a vision of him exercising; he wouldn't have run from a hive of angry bees. When he came home from his job, he wasn't looking for the running shoes that he did not own. He was looking for his recliner. He turned the news on, ate a lidfull of Planter's Peanuts, put his feet up and maybe had a gin and tonic.

It's not clear to me whether he considered exercise unnecessary, or unobtainable; or, like most men of his generation, he just never considered it. He worked for a living: why would he exercise?

Fortunately, those attitudes are changing. We've come to understand that a life of leisure is unhealthy and that any activity is good activity. Although the age-related declines in fitness capacity can be discouraging, note that some of those losses are simply related to inactivity. The body is miserly: it does not send resources to muscles that are not being used (see the Move It or Lose It chapter).

So although any activity is good, exercise is better.

Why Intensity Matters

The difference between being active and exercising is a matter of intensity. For a variety of reasons, intensity matters.

When it comes to cardiovascular fitness, performing hours of low-demand exercise doesn't really improve one's aerobic fitness. You cannot improve your VO2 max without pushing your heart to do more than it is used to doing. This is why the latest guidelines for aerobic exercise recommend shorter periods of moderate to vigorous intensity, ones that increase the heart rate anywhere from 55 percent to 90 percent of its maximum.

In a world where many of us feel starved for time, this move towards briefer but more intense workouts is a welcome change. Stationary bikes and treadmills that climb imaginary but very 'real' hills have made it easier than ever to break a sweat rather than just keep the hamster wheel turning. A 10K run in 60 minutes is certainly not unhealthy per se, but it might not be as beneficial as a 5K run in 25 minutes. Besides, longer and slower runs can eat up time and our enthusiasm without adding additional cardiovascular benefits.

This is one of the reasons that a marathon isn't necessarily the healthiest endeavor. I've run a couple. They are punishing. They are painful. To be sure, they are a pinnacle of discipline, dedication, and athletic achievement, but there may be healthier ways to accomplish those things.

Similarly, when it comes to strength training, intensity matters. Multiple sets of low-weight exercises don't really improve muscle strength. The reason has to do with how muscle is built. On a microscopic level, putting strain on a muscle causes some of its fibers to tear. This is the soreness that you feel after a workout. These muscle fibers are then rebuilt, remodeled, and become stronger and larger. Bones, too, grow thicker where lines of force are applied—which is why zero-gravity of space leads to thinning bones, and why weight bearing exercises (as opposed to swimming, or being on a bike) build stronger bones.

Calisthenics can certainly improve flexibility, but your biceps won't get stronger by simply flexing your arm repetitively. The bicep muscle needs to contract against resistance to do that, hence the term "resistance training," where weights, exercise tubing, or your own weight provide that critical resistance. Think of the difference between walking and walking up stairs. On stairs, our legs are bearing much more weight, much more resistance. One can walk for miles, but one can't walk miles of stairs.

Because intensity matters, groups like the American College of Sports Medicine suggest weightlifting regimens that are shorter in terms of reps, but more challenging in terms of weight.

Where to Start or Restart Your New Life as an AARPathlete?

Here's an amalgamation of what most guidelines recommend:

Moderate Intensity Exercise: 2.5–5 hours per week

You *could* cram your week's allotment of exercise into one day, if you're task oriented and can't wait to cross things off your list. But you'll be healthier and have fewer injuries if you spread it out over two or more days. As I mentioned earlier, there are additional health benefits beyond the five-hour mark, but you might be too tired to care.

Moderate-Vigorous, or Straight Vigorous Intensity Exercise: 2.5–1.25 hours per week

I have to remind myself that there is still some math that I can do without a calculator. Here one can see that at 1.25 hrs/wk, a vigorous intensity workout is half as long as a moderate one of 2.5 hrs/wk. Or—and I am not just showing off here—that a moderate workout is twice as long as a vigorous one.

Muscle-Strengthening Activities of Moderate or Greater Intensity Two or More Times a Week

These should involve all major muscle groups (arm, forearm, thigh, leg, spinal muscles, and abdominal muscles) and you should go to the point where you feel it would be difficult to do another repetition (generally, 8 to 12 reps).

However one chooses to exercise, remember to maintain good form and posture. Twisting and turning to get those last couple reps in is asking small muscle groups to do more than they should. As most of us experienced in the high school social scene, it's possible to diminish yourself by trying too hard.

I am a doctor, not a life coach or a fitness trainer. Find a professional if you need one. But here are a few suggestions as you attempt to sing the body electric:

- Avoid deadlines and all-or-nothing ultimatums. Most human progress is made in fits and spurts. Try and try again.
- Forgive yourself for the weeks that got away from you. This will happen. You don't want life to be the death of you.
- If you've never been big on working out, it may take months or years to really change. Habits—even good ones—are hard to break because they've been ingrained over time. So it may take some time to develop a sustainable exercise ethic. It may take some time psychologically for you to recognize the guy who is lifting weights, or the guy who is sweating it out on a stationary bike that looks like a prop from a futuristic movie.
- If you're interested in geeking out on this workout intensity stuff, consider a lifetime subscription to The Adult Compendi-

um of Physical Activities, a free website designed by Arizona State University. The compendium provides Metabolic Equivalent of Task (MET) data on all kinds of activities. If you go to the Activity Categories tab and then scroll down to 13—Self Care, you'll find that "sitting on toilet, eliminating while standing or squatting" will run you 1.8 METs, while "having hair or nails done by someone else, sitting" is just 1.3. In the 4—Fishing and Hunting category, "hunting, flying fox, squirrel" is 3.0 METs and "hunting, deer, elk, large game" is a 6.0. That rises to 11.3 METs if you have to drag the carcass back to the truck. In the 1—Bicycling category, "unicycling" is 5.0 METs, and in 10—Music Playing, playing the "trombone, standing," is 3.5 METs. This is life-altering stuff that raises endless questions, such as:

1. How many METs would it be to drag a carcass out of the woods on a unicycle? 2. Or have your hair done while playing the trombone?

Isn't Exercise a Young Man's Sport? Isn't It Hard on Joints?

When I was growing up, gyms were only found in schools and bigger churches, not in every strip mall or people's homes. Exercise training was what one did to participate in a sport, and sports (save men's softball, oddly enough) were for kids. The line on strenuous exercise and athletic training (anything more than a brisk walk) for adult men and women was that it was either unnecessary ("I'm not playing a sport, so why should I be training for one," "I already work for a living") or that, with advancing age, they were simply too frail for it. They'd just end up hurting themselves.

This relationship between perceived frailty and risk of injury is a kind of self-fulfilling prophecy. To avoid injury or a heart attack, you might talk yourself into avoiding anything but low-intensity exercise, which then leaves you more prone to the very things you were looking to avoid: injury and heart disease. The truth is that when anyone *of any age* is out of shape and tries to exert themselves, the risk of injury is higher. It's certainly true that older folks take longer to recover from

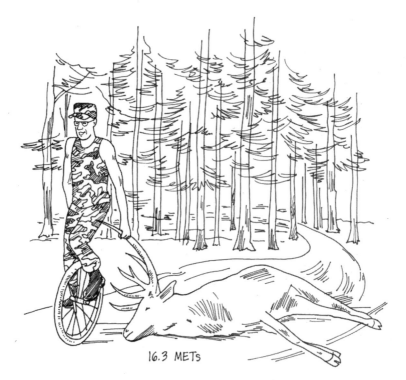

16.3 METs

injury—muscle fibers torn with strengthening exercises can heal in two weeks for the youthful, and a month for the not-so-youthful.

One frequently voiced concern is that more aggressive exercise could end up wearing out one's joints and lead to arthritis. That idea holds up to some commonsense scrutiny: the screen door hinge has only so many turns in it before the repetitive movements abrade the metal and the hinge loosens up, which only accelerates the wear.

Like the door, our joints are mechanical in nature, but unlike the door, our joints are alive. The living "connective tissue" of our bones, ligaments, tendons, and cartilage are in a perpetual state of remodeling, and they respond to stresses (rather miraculously) by increasing that remodeling, bulking up in areas where extra heft is needed.

So regular exercise—even intense exercise—is good for our joints. The increased risk for osteoarthritis that comes with participating in sports is thought to be due to either a single-impact kind of disaster (the fall onto the shoulder, the weirdly twisted knee), or to a series of smaller-impact disasters (so-called "dings," as in "I dinged up my shoulder playing sand volleyball"), and not due to regular use.

There is one way in which the door-hinge analogy does hold up: our joints are indeed mechanical, and they work the best when alignments are optimal. Injury comes most easily at the extremes of position, when the joint is misaligned and not in a good position to handle a load. This is why body mechanics and ergonomics are so important, particularly for a patient with low-back pain who needs to lift a weight. Muscle strength is also critical, because muscles are important in maintaining proper joint mechanics. For example, quadriceps strength is critical to knee stability. Flexibility helps to maintain posture and joint mechanics too.

Getting Started

1. Heart Check

If you've never really been serious about exercise, or only been serious about avoiding it, it makes sense to start with a visit to your doctor.

The primary emphasis should be on the cardiovascular system, looking for coronary artery disease that might not have given you any trouble during your storied fantasy football career, but could be a problem under the rigors of racing your obsessively lean, ultra-competitive daughter-in-law to the tape. You can live with sore muscles if you overdo it on the weights, but a "sore" heart has the potential to put you facedown in the bushes, where you or a passerby are unlikely to find a CPR defibrillator kit. Depending on your age and risk factors, further testing might be in order (see the Heart Disease Prevention chapter).

Doctor or no doctor, here's the good news: having a heart attack during a workout is a very rare event. According to the 2008 Physical Activity Guidelines for Americans, "Inactive people who gradually progress over time to relatively moderate-intensity activity have no known risk of sudden cardiac events and very low risk of bone, muscle, or joint injuries."

2. Workout Clothing as a Motivational Tool

Assuming you get the all-clear from your doctor or loved ones, go out and buy a closet full of expensive athletic clothing and footwear, as this cements the commitment: you're going to *have* to get in shape to justify the cost of buying that stuff. Particularly the neon-colored stuff, or the tights that coddle your 'junk' in a way that makes those around you visibly uncomfortable.

3. If You're Just Starting, "Start Low and Go Slow"

The key is gradual progression. If you're starting from nothing— physiologic Ground Zero—start with light-intensity activities such as walking, or very casually hunting flying foxes with a trombone. This will help you avoid the archetypal New Year's Eve fitness resolution debacle, an ephemeral shooting-star experience that often flashes out by February or March because an overly enthusiastic January led to excessive soreness and injury.

Take as long as you need to ramp things up. If the last sweat-drenching experience you had was in a college racquetball class, then you might need some time to feel comfortable that breathing that hard or having your heart go that fast isn't going to break something. One of the 'gifts' of aging is having to fret about things that you didn't used to worry about. When I was doing wind sprints in high school basketball and there didn't seem to be nearly enough oxygen in the room, I never thought to myself, "I wonder if I'm having a heart attack."

Acknowledging that exercise is a very uncommon trigger for heart attacks, and that most occur at rest, keep this in mind: the shortness of breath, sweatiness, and chest wall pain/soreness/tightness caused by vigorous chest wall expansion during exercise should resolve fairly quickly with rest. If it does not, then there might be something more serious going on.

Shouldn't I Be Enjoying This?

Endorphins (the brain's Oreo cookie reward system) vary person to person, but for me, strenuous exercise—pushing myself to run/pedal/swim/jump/climb *hard*—is not pleasurable. It does not feel immediately rewarding. It feels immediately taxing. There are days when I come home from work and exercising is the last thing on my priority list. I robotically force myself forward: "Put on shorts; put on T-shirt; tie on running shoes; walk out door; start feigned running motion." It takes effort and drive to stay with it, and sometimes the biggest push to go fast through a workout is to have it over with. For me, the reward generally comes when the workout is over—and includes a sense of physical flushing (a relaxing, hot tub sensation), stress reduction, and a feeling of accomplishment. I sleep better that night, too.

Oddly enough, for me, Nordic (cross-country) skiing is an exception to the rule of strenuous exercise being strenuously difficult. Despite its demands (Nordic skiers and triathletes tend to have very high VO2 max), I find it immediately invigorating. I want to go fast. Fast is fun. May you find your own equivalent.

Injuries: Recovering the Satellites

There must be a name for a negative milestone—how about a "millstone"—and one millstone that almost everyone experiences is the first time you injure yourself and then slowly come to the realization that this thing isn't ever going to heal up and return to normal. You never actually considered yourself invincible, but hey, this was the general message life had been giving you throughout your young and supple and quickly regenerative years.

For me, this millstone occurred in college, when I was out skiing and wrenched my thumb backward in a way that geometry and anatomy cannot reconcile. It got better, slowly, but as weeks turned to months, it was clear that it was never going back to normal. The injury put all of my athletic endeavors into a different light: maybe putting myself into harm's way for, say, a critical rebound in a pickup basketball game at the YMCA was not a good long-term health investment.

Other injuries followed, of course, as did the realization that healing seemed to take longer as I grew older. Muscle fibers rely on what are termed "satellite cells" to make needed repairs. These cells sit around the periphery of a muscle but spring into action when injury occurs and muscle fibers needs to be rebuilt. Satellite cells are important in strength training, since muscle-building exercises induce microtrauma (shredding of existing fiber), which causes muscles to be rebuilt and enhanced. As we age, the number of satellite cells decreases, and—you guessed it—they don't function as well. They shag balls like an old Mariano Rivera. They retire and take jobs up in the broadcast booth.

If you do become injured, and you probably will, because you are alive after all, the usual applies: rest, ice, elevation, and pain control. So-called "Nonsteroidal anti-inflammatory drugs" (NSAIDS) are helpful for the pain and inflammation that comes with injury. Ibuprofen, "Vitamin I" as it's sometimes called, is the most well-known drug in the NSAID class, and naproxen is probably second. These medications work well and are generally well tolerated if taken for a few days here and there; but they do have their own risks, as I detailed in the Low Back Pain chapter. The list of side effects for any drug is the same whether you're age 21 or 71, but the 71-year-old is more likely to experience them and have more trouble dealing with them. So be careful.

Acetaminophen (Tylenol) is not an NSAID, but it can be an effective pain reliever, and it doesn't have the heart, stomach and kidney issues that "Vitamin I" and the rest of the NSAID gang do. It can, however, cause liver damage if used in excess, so follow the dosing directions.

There are a few situations in which NSAIDs can be bad medicine. In certain types of tendonitis or in stress fractures, NSAIDs can sometimes retard healing. NSAIDs should not be used to reduce the pain just so you can train through an acute injury, you idiot! The pain is trying to tell you something—primarily, "Knock it off." Most injuries will require either stopping or backing off from your usual training regimen.

But you should stay active if at all possible. As any middle-aged athlete like me (with heavyweight sponsors like Jerry's Home Medical Equipment and The International NSAID Institute) will tell you, it doesn't take long to lose the conditioning you built up prior to the injury.

SEXERCISE

What Are the Cardiovascular Demands of This Ancient Ritual, and Could It Kill You?

I miss those heady days of the early 2000s, when Pecker Power drugs like Viagra and Cialis were major sponsors of the nightly news and every major sporting event. The ads were richly entertaining (a cacophony of muscle cars, rock bands, and, yes, claw-foot bathtubs!) and it was often difficult to tell whether they were satirizing or sanctifying the nobility of the aging male.

Gone but not forgotten, the erectile dysfunction drug ads of yore left viewers wondering about a more serious and potentially troubling issue, a kind of sideways disclaimer: "Ask your doctor if you're healthy enough for sexual activity."

Healthy enough? Had sex suddenly become like high school sports, with participants needing a physical from their doctors and a permission slip from their parents? But the question—and the seed of fear—had been planted: what are the cardiovascular demands of sex, and how risky is it? Indeed, anyone who's ever experienced *extreme twitterpation* can appreciate what a heart-thumping event sex can be. The Elizabethan expression for sexual climax—"I died in your arms"—comes to mind.

Honestly, I had no idea how to answer the "healthy enough for sex" question if my patients were to ask it, and a quick survey of my physician colleagues showed they didn't

MAN OVERBOARD!

Sex is not that physically rigorous—categorized as light-to-moderate exertion. Like climbing two flights of stairs in 10 seconds, though more interesting. It does increase the risk of having a heart attack by a very small margin, but what a way to go.

either. "Give them a stress test...?" was the most frequent reply, the pitch of their voices rising through the sentence, indicating their befuddlement.

Sex under the Microscope (It's Cramped in Here)

As you might imagine (but frankly, I hope you haven't), it's not easy to find research volunteers willing to have intercourse in a lab setting, with researchers "monitoring things" and with all the wires and monitors running here and there. Besides, it's become increasingly more difficult to find funding for this kind of basic "bench research"—doing studies that may answer important clinical questions but that don't have a new pill or a potion to be sold if the research works out. There needs to be a financial carrot, even if it is bent.

So, there's not been a lot of research into this area, and the studies are small. But what can they tell us?

The most basic way to measure someone's cardiovascular output is by monitoring blood pressure and pulse rate. A classic treadmill stress test does exactly that, monitoring blood pressure, pulse, and the electrical activity of the heart while the participant walks on a quickening and steepening treadmill. They are encouraged to go until they feel spent.

A 2007 study in the *American Journal of Cardiology* put a group of 30 men and women in their early to mid fifties through a treadmill test. Then they sent the participants home with a blood pressure and pulse monitoring device they could wear during intercourse. Pulse monitoring was continuous, and blood pressure was recorded every six minutes; male participants were asked to activate a blood pressure reading when they reached the "Surrender Dorothy!" climax.

Researchers found that sexual activity, measured from foreplay through S.D.! lasted about 30 minutes, and participants pooped out on the treadmill test after about 11 minutes. That's almost certainly because few if any people find a stress test to be pleasurable, and because the treadmill was much more physically intense. For men, average maximum heart rates reached during sex were 72 percent of what they hit on the treadmill; the number was 64 percent for women. Using another measure—heart rate × blood pressure—the cardiovascular

SURRENDER DOROTHY

2.5 ~ 3.3 METs

peak of sex for the men was about 7 METs of exertion (1 MET being the amount of energy expended while sitting quietly in place). For the women it was 5 METs. The differences between the sexes could be due to techniques or positioning, which the researchers said were none of our business.

Those MET numbers put hanky-panky into the moderate-exertion category, although as the researchers pointed out, those exertion levels are sustained for a very short period of time. When the smoke runs out of the witch's broom, the witch comes crashing to the ground in seconds.

Treadmill testing can tell us a lot about someone's cardiovascular fitness, but the high point of fitness testing typically includes adding a face mask to measure how much oxygen the participant is using. A 1984 study managed to do just that, recruiting 10 married couples (average age 33) to have intercourse in a monitored lab setting. (For unclear reasons, the women in this study went unmonitored.) The oxygen-measuring mask, researchers noted, did limit physical expression such as kissing and talking (though some of the male participants may have found this to be more of a convenience than a limitation).

After checking baseline vitals, participants were given a perfunctory five-minute period of foreplay and then told to prepare for liftoff. The process was repeated in four different permutations: man on top, woman on top, non-coital stimulation of man by woman, and man stimulating self. As if these brave men of science didn't have enough to do—donating their bodies to research and all—each was also asked to signal the start and end of his climax by activating a handheld event-marker button that served as a kind of checkered flag.

Not surprisingly, the lab setting and all the monitoring was a real mood killer: foreplay to *S.D.!* lasted about 11 minutes.

The data showed that foreplay created small increases in cardiac and metabolic expenditures, but the big surge of effort came during the 10 to 16 seconds it took, on average, to achieve orgasm. When the man was on top, he spent an average of 3.3 METs on coitus; with the woman on top, he used just 2.5 METs. Meanwhile, stimulation-via-partner and the do-it-yourself method expended only 1.7 METs. Researchers found a fair amount of variability among the different couples. For example, one man expended 2.0 METs and another 5.4, proving that, like most things, sex is different for everybody.

Gigolos Demoted to "Non-Athlete" Status

The results of these kinds of studies have pushed gigolos out of the ranks of professional athletes and placed sexercise on the border between "light-intensity" (1.1 to 2.9 METs) and "moderate-intensity" (3.0 to 5.9 METs) exertion. This puts the rigor of sexual activity somewhere between light-intensity activities such as a *stroll around the office* (2.0), *washing the dishes* or *playing the guitar* (2.0 to 2.5), and a *game of darts* (2.5) and moderate-intensity forays, such as *cleaning out the garage* (3.0), *cartless golfing* (4.3), *general carpentry* (3.6), *fishing from riverbank and walking* (4.0), and *walking at a brisk 4 mph* (5.0).

Since one man's *carrying and stacking wood* (5.5) might be another man's *mowing the lawn with a walk-behind power mower* (5.5), a more standardized and reproducible comparison equates the exertion of sexual activity with *walking a mile in 15 to 20 minutes* or *climbing two flights of stairs in 10 seconds*. If those sorts of activities are beyond your physical reach or bring on shortness of breath or chest heaviness—symptoms suggestive of coronary artery disease—then you *really should* ask your doctor if you're healthy enough for sexual activity.

So, whatever it *feels* like, sex is a brief and not particularly strenuous endeavor. Although there are exceptions (and you, kind reader, are undoubtedly one of them), sex becomes less physiologically intense as we age. It might remain just as pleasurable, but it inevitably becomes less vigorous, even for the likes of "The Godfather of Fitness" Jack LaLanne, who in his nineties claimed, without prompting (or even encouragement, really), that he could still "put a smile" on his wife's face.

One caveat: the cardiovascular demands of sex could be higher in certain circumstances, because sex can be an extremely emotional event, and emotions can vary. (Note that the two studies I mentioned included those with stable and familiar sex partners.) As the term "casual sex" suggests, the who, where, and why components around intercourse can radically alter the physical demands of the act. Emotional arousal triggers the release of adrenaline, which has potent effects on blood pressure and pulse. Sex researchers Masters and Johnson proved that in the 1960s, observing that the intensity of the physiologic response to sex was proportional to the degree of sexual tension/attraction.

Can a Roll in the Hay Turn into a Long Dirt Nap?

So we know that sexercise gives you a brief light-to-moderate workout, but could it lead to a heart attack?

The answer is yes, but don't panic! The risk of having a heart attack *goes up two-and-a-half times in the two-hour period following sexual activity.* That sounds like a big increase, but if you double the risk of an uncommon event it's still going to be an uncommon event. Walking through a zoo quadruples your risk of being attacked by a lion, from one in a billion to four in a billion.

In the end, sexercise increases one's real-life 'absolute risk' of a heart attack by an infinitesimally small amount, because the baseline risk is very small and most men aren't continuously having sex. If one has sex once a week, that 2-hour window of increased risk adds up to 100 hours—out of the 8,760 hours that make up a year. That's why a once-a-week sexcapade increases the risk of a heart attack over a year's time by just 0.01% for low-risk individuals and by 0.1% for higher-risk individuals.

Doctors understand that most heart attacks occur because an atherosclerotic scar inside one of the coronary arteries splits open, triggering a blood clot that then closes off the entire blood vessel. Things like smoking, diabetes, and high blood pressure lead to atherosclerotic buildup, but it's not clear what specifically triggers the acute rupture and subsequent heart attack. Certain behaviors do seem more likely than others to set off an unfortunate episode: waking up in the morning, physical exertion, sexual activity, and anger. Yet all of these taken together can only account for a minority of cases. Physical (but non-sexual) overexertion is thought to cause about 5 percent of all heart attacks, anger 3 percent, and sex less than 1 percent.

It's worth noting that although sex and anger—different forms of extreme emotional arousal—increase the risk of a heart attack risk about two and a half times, anger is a far more common trigger because people have more angry outbursts than they do sex.

If the risk of having a heart attack during intercourse is so very *small*, why make such a *big* deal about it in the ads? The Food and Drug Administration's Division of Drug Marketing, Advertising, and Communications stipulates that broadcast ads must include the drug's most important risks, and having a heart attack whilst flying your broomstick over the Emerald City qualifies as such. Like passing out skateboards to nursing home residents, the FDA must have felt that medication designed to bring older men out of sexual retirement was promoting risky behavior.

What about a stress test? If you're not having chest pain doing moderate-intensity activities, such as *sweeping floors or carpet, vacuuming, mopping* (3.0 to 3.5 METs), you're probably fine. If you want reassurance, you could try pushing into the vigorous-intensity category by *shoveling sand, coal, etc.* (7.0 METs). Or talk with your doctor. We're less befuddled about this topic now.

The lesson here is that having sex increases one's risk of having a heart attack, but only to a very small degree, and let's be honest: everything increases one's risk for something. Standing increases the risk of falling. Eating increases the risk of choking.

Whatever you do, avoid mixing physical exertion, anger, and sex. It's a formula that works for many of the dis-reality shows out there, but don't try it at home.

14 RISKY BUSINESS

Let's Get Serious: A Fear-Focused Approach to Better Health

Okay, you're more than halfway through *Man Overboard!* Congratulations!

We tackled your sitty disposition, aching back, and receding hairline. We embarked on a magical mystery tour through the shadowy worlds of low testosterone, sexercise, and sleep, and we've shown how swapping French fries for alpine turds can jump-start both your metabolism and your fledgling career as a celebrated AARPathlete.

We had some fun, but from here on out the road gets a little steeper, as we embrace a fear-focused approach to better health. Let me explain.

Fear isn't such a bad thing—if it's focused and proportionate to the threat. Ideally, our sense of fear should be firmly lashed to the actual level of risk involved. Except humans are pretty bad at evaluating risk. Fear is an emotion, and emotion tends to cloud logical thinking.

We walk into the undulating ocean surf, feeling fully alive and vaca-

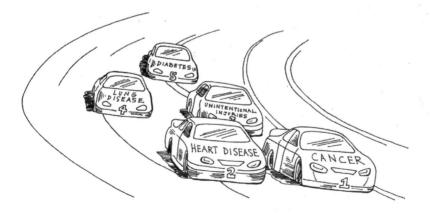

tional, the warm salty air sitting heavy on our skin. And then, suddenly, the thought of being attacked by a shark puts a lump in the throat and a tightening in the scrotum, even though the most dangerous part of your entire day was the drive to the beach.

Here in landlocked Minnesota, we're short on saltwater and sharks, but we now have a healthy wolf population in the northern part of the state. A walk in the northwoods, if interrupted by the sound or even the thought of this most capable carnivore, brings goose pimples and a quickening pace, even though no human being has ever been killed by a wolf. Bears yes, and we have plenty of those. Wolves no.

So, as we settle into the third half of *Man Overboard!* (fun fact: 5 out of every 4 Americans don't really understand fractions), let's think clearly about what we aging males are really up against, so that our health fears are in line with our actual health risks.

What we are *not* up against is zebras (unless, I suppose, you are reading this on safari). There's an expression in medicine about "chasing zebras," and it has nothing to do with striped horses, or referee apparel, or life on the Serengeti plains. It's the penchant that doctors (and patients) sometimes have for obsessing over the possibility of impossibly rare, bizarre diagnoses. There is an allure in the fantastical that does not exist in the routine.

But common things are common, and when it comes to one's health, you'll be far better off focusing on the humdrum health problems that are most likely to come your way, rather than the list of illnesses that came up on an episode of *The Office*. After Dwight had ransacked the employee health plan, Jim submitted the following maladies for insurance coverage: leprosy, flesh-eating bacteria, hot dog fingers, government-created killer-nano-robot infections, Count Choculitis, an inverted penis.

So in that spirit, let's take a serious look at the CDC's "10 Leading Causes of Death in the United States," focusing on males, of all races, over the last two decades.

Unintentional (i.e. accidental) injury is the leading cause of death in men until they reach their mid-forties, where it takes third place till age 65, and moves to the sixth, then seventh spot thereafter.

The three heavy hitters in this accidental injury category are car crashes, falls, and "poisonings" –typically due to overdoses of illegal or prescription drugs, but also including alcohol, pesticides, or carbon monoxide. For young male drivers, motor vehicle accidents cause 60% of accidental deaths, but that percentage levels off to around 30% until geezerhood. Deaths from drug overdose make up nearly 50% of accidental deaths in men ages 25-55 but fall sharply thereafter. Death by gravity—falling—is a very minor issue until we hit our mid-50's, where it's responsible for 13% of unintentional deaths. The risk rises rapidly thereafter—to 30% for men age 65-74, and 60% for older men—which is why two of the *Man Overboard! Keynote Sponsors*™ are LeafGuard and the CDC's *Take Away His Ladder!* campaign.

If you're looking to live a long and *active* life, you might be concerned about disability. The most severe form of disability—wherein one can no longer be truly independent—is most commonly due to spinal cord injuries (causing paraplegia or quadriplegia) and strokes.

Eighty percent of spinal cord injuries occur in men, and the causes often fall into the "Ooh, shouldn't have done that" category. Interestingly, the average age of injury has slowly risen to 42, an age when you'd think we'd know better.

The point is, it doesn't make a lot of sense to perseverate about your cholesterol level, or your body fat percentage, or shaving a few seconds off your 10K personal best if you're driving while impaired (alcohol, drugs, sleep depravation or *texting*), not wearing a seat belt, using a picnic table to extend your ladder, or bouldering with friends and getting in way over your head.

In other types of accidental disasters, gun violence ranks pretty high. Aside from hunting accidents, this has more to do with unaddressed public health and economic disparities (having no other option than to live in a dangerous place) than personal health choices.

While *Man Overboard!* does not have a chapter on strokes, they, too, are something to be feared. In the hospital where I work, patients can be teetering on the edge of death and undergo very complex surgeries or procedures, but most recover and go home. They may be weak and stiff and sore, but those things are temporary. And yet a stroke— the death of a relatively small but critical portion of brain tissue—has the potential to leave a person permanently altered, unable to walk, talk, eat, toilet themselves, or even swallow. Because the risk factors for stroke are generally the same as those for heart disease, we'll discuss them in the aptly titled chapter Heart Disease Prevention.

Although there is an appealing simplicity in worrying about *everything*, the focus of our final chapters will be on the most likely causes of morbidity and mortality—that's cardiovascular disease and cancer. From age 45 on, those two sit atop the leaderboard for cause of death.

Let's make the most important things the most important things, so we can stop worrying and get on with enjoying our lives. If you develop something rare, like Count Choculitis or hot dog fingers, you can certainly make an appointment with Dr. Dwight Schrute, assuming he's in-network for your health insurance plan and your approach to health care aligns with his. Which seems unlikely.

> What did I do? I did my job. I slashed benefits to the bone; I saved this company money. Was I too harsh? Maybe. I don't believe in coddling people; in the wild, there is no health care. In the wild, health care is, "Ow, I hurt my leg; I can't run; a lion eats me and I'm dead."
> —*Dr. Dwight Schrute*, The Office

HEART DISEASE
Elephants, Whac-a-Moles, Metaphor Malpractice, and the Soothing Effects of Statins

After age 45, heart disease roars to the front of the "AARP Motor Speedway's *Race to the Death*" for men, dueling for the lead position with cancer until it finally takes the checkered flag.

When doctors talk about heart disease, they're typically talking about coronary artery disease—blockage of the arteries that supply the heart muscle with blood. Of course, there are all kinds of bad things that can happen to a heart, but in this chapter we'll stick to coronary artery disease and leave heart failure, heart valve problems, and electrical issues like atrial fibrillation for the hair-raising sequel, *Man Overboard! 2: The Avengers Enroll in Medicare.*

It's a little counterintuitive to think that an organ that is literally a sack full of blood would need its own blood supply, but it does, and the right and left coronary arteries course down the outside of the heart, feeding the heart muscle from the outside in. If that supply becomes substantially blocked, the heart muscle downstream from the blockage can be either injured or killed, depending on how severe the reduction in blood flow was, and how long the shortage lasted.

Every year more than a million Americans find themselves in their local emergency room with some or all of the hall-

MAN OVERBOARD!

Coronary blockage #1 killer. Inflammation and injury lead to scarring that plugs arteries. Stress tests find only big plaques, but small plaques can cause BIG problems. Angioplasty with stents are best for active, serious blockages. Medications and treating risk factors are best preventive therapy.

mark symptoms of coronary disease: shortness of breath; pain in the chest, jaw, left shoulder, or left arm; nausea; or a heavy, suffocating chest pressure that is often described as feeling like an elephant has plopped down on the victim's chest. Which always raises the question, with so many large animals to demonize, why choose the docile and intelligent elephant?

Whatever the metaphorical source of the chest pain and pressure—elephant, black rhino, Budweiser Clydesdale—this symptom is called "angina." If the heart muscle ends up dying, it's called a "heart attack" or "myocardial infarction" (MI for short). Sometimes you'll hear the phrase "He had a coronary," or if you're from New England, "He had a car'nary."

A "Can't-Miss Diagnosis"

At the risk of getting too technical, some heart attacks are big and some are small. Regardless of the size of the attack, the most serious immediate risk is that the damaged heart muscle will trigger a lethal arrhythmia, causing the heart to quiver rather than beat, which, at the risk of getting too technical, is a serious-shit problem—a "cardiac arrest." With the pump quivering rather than contracting, there is now zero blood flow to the heart, not to mention the rest of the organs.

For too many people, a cardiac arrest is the first sign that they have coronary disease: half of those who die from a cardiac arrest didn't know they even had heart problems. They maybe had some mild chest symptoms—perhaps a little indigestion, or a five-pound cashmere lop-eared bunny rabbit sitting on the chest—followed by an arrhythmia that brought them tumbling, unconscious, to the floor. This is why we take heart disease so seriously: it can be immediately lethal in a way that few other diseases are, making it a can't-miss diagnosis.

Fortunately, some people with coronary disease do get recognizable warning signs because their blockages develop slowly. Their angina symptoms first begin appearing at the end of exercise or routine activities and are quickly relieved with a little rest. Over some period of time the angina comes on sooner (20 minutes into one's 35-minute workout routine, or halfway out to the mailbox); it takes less exertion to trigger them and more rest to make the pain or shortness of breath go away. With a little time for introspection, these lucky folks can recognize what's happening and get evaluated. Plus, if atherosclerosis arises slowly, the heart muscle downstream from the blockage can adjust to the decreased blood flow. It can learn to get by with less. Or the heart can even develop what we call "collateral blood flow." If your fingers were blood vessels, and your ring finger was getting slowly blocked, imagine your pinky and middle finger slowly getting bigger to make up the difference. Magic!

We don't understand why for some patients, coronary artery disease shows up like the in-laws—suddenly and without warning—while others get plenty of forewarning. But we're getting better at finding disease earlier. We'll talk about that later in this chapter, and also in the chapter on heart disease prevention. For now, let's take a look at what a diseased coronary artery looks like, and how it got that way.

Metaphor Malpractice: Your Pipes Aren't Clogged—They're Inflamed

For decades, the public and even the scientific view of atherosclerosis was that it was a plumbing problem. Cholesterol builds up and clogs arteries the way too much toilet paper clogs the toilet. Cholesterol medications like Lipitor provide a little Drano action. Angioplasty—ballooning open the areas narrowed by globs of cholesterol—is the medical version of the Roto-Rooter, and open-heart bypass surgery is a bigger project, like putting in new pipes to go around the old ones that have become blocked.

As tidy and familiar as this plumbing metaphor might be (who among us hasn't wielded the mighty plunger?), it prevented us from understanding the true nature of atherosclerosis. That's a 15-yard penalty for metaphor malpractice, and unscientific-like conduct.

Yes, the coronary arteries do become clogged, but that's a secondary issue. The primary driver of all forms of atherosclerosis is inflammation: smoking, diabetes, high blood pressure, and bad cholesterol scour the delicate inner lining of the arteries (called the "intima"), causing inflammation and then scars that we call "plaques."

These plaques aren't just an inanimate wad of toilet paper (or *somebody's* discarded Happy Meal toy) causing a physical, mechanical obstruction. They are alive, contain several different types of cells, and exist in various levels of growth and irritation. When a plaque becomes so swollen and inflamed that it ruptures, the ragged exposed surface attracts a blood clot. Suddenly a coronary artery that was 30 percent blocked is now 100 percent blocked—30 percent by plaque and 70 percent by blood clot. This is the most common way for a heart attack to develop.

Well, so what? Metaphors, you say, are mind candy for English majors and literary types. The problem with this plumbing view of coronary artery disease is that it skewed our sense of what this disease really is and the best way to treat it. To add another metaphor (I am an English major), building codes, smoke detectors, and fire trucks all fight fires; but the first two are preventative therapy, and fire trucks are symptomatic therapy. For a while there, we went a little crazy with our fire trucks, at the expense of smoke detectors. Read on.

Angiograms, Angioplasty, Stents, and Problems #1, 2, and 3

If you show up in the emergency room with a wildebeest on your chest, sooner or later you'll likely end up getting a coronary angiogram. If the wildebeest feeling is signaling a serious heart attack, you might get wheeled away for one in a matter of minutes.

Long considered the gold standard test for finding coronary artery blockages, a coronary angiogram is a procedure that entails threading a small catheter (doctors describe all catheters as "small") through an artery in the arm or groin and then up into the coronary arteries. A solution called "contrast" is injected through the catheter to make the inside of the arteries appear dark on X-ray. A healthy artery looks smooth and wide open, like a tree—a larger trunk splitting off into smaller branches. A diseased artery looks narrowed and beaded—or in the most severe cases, completely blocked, giving the appearance that a branch of the tree was lopped off.

In the early days of cardiology, an angiogram was only diagnostic—if a blockage was found, it was dealt with either by using medications, or by coronary artery bypass graft surgery. "Bypass surgery" entails running a small bone saw (doctors describe all bone saws as "small") through the sternum to expose the heart. Veins from the leg or an artery from the chest are then used to reroute, i.e. bypass, blood flow around the blockage(s). This works well, but it's pretty violent and carries some serious surgical risks.

Looking to offer a less invasive treatment option than bypass surgery, cardiologists invented a procedure called "angioplasty." If significant blockages were noted on angiogram, a small (in this case, it really is small, believe me) balloon is inflated inside the blockage, stretching open the plaque and reversing the blockage. This also worked, but too often the ballooned area would, in a matter of days to weeks, col-

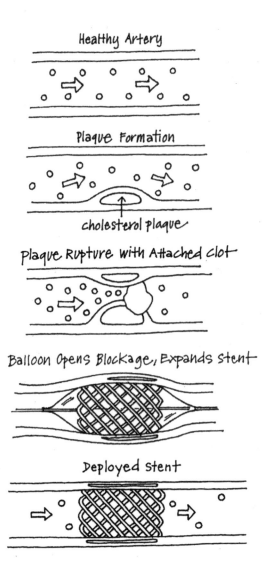

Healthy Artery

Plaque Formation

cholesterol plaque

Plaque Rupture with Attached clot

Balloon Opens Blockage, Expands stent

Deployed stent

lapse back in on itself and reblock the artery. This problem, which we'll call Problem #1, led to the invention of the coronary artery stent, a short wire-mesh straw that could be slipped into the ballooned area to keep it from collapsing.

Stents worked well, except for Problem #2: sometimes the stent would trigger overaggressive scar formation, reblocking the artery. So the solution to Problem #2 was to coat the stents with a substance that prevented the scarring process. These are called "drug-eluting stents," but because no one has ever heard of the word "elute," they are often referred to as "coated stents." Practically speaking, these are the only kind of stents we use nowadays.

This approach worked well except for Problem #3: coated stents have a penchant for attracting blood clots so patients need to be on an additional blood-thinning drug for six months at a minimum. This seemed to work. And on the seventh day, the cardiologist rested.

Whac-a-Mole Cardiology

But on the eighth day she got back to work. Armed with this much less invasive alternative to bypass surgery, it seemed like any sizeable coronary blockage could and probably should be stented. It was Whac-a-Mole cardiology, and you won the game by banging the head of whatever atherosclerotic plaque stuck its head out of the hole. Coronary catheterization labs were popping up everywhere, like Krispy Kreme donut franchises.

Though the results of a successful angioplasty were technically miraculous—an artery went from 70 percent to 0 percent blocked—there was mounting evidence that the clinical benefits were less impressive for some patients. A 2007 study in the *New England Journal of Medicine* randomized a group of patients presenting with coronary artery disease and "chronic stable angina" (where angina comes rarely or briefly, or at predictable levels of exertion) to be treated either with medications, or angioplasty followed by medications. The study found that although angioplasty lowered their odds of needing to be readmitted to the hospital with chest pain in the future, all the more serious outcomes—death, heart attack, and stroke—seemed unchanged.

MAN OVERBOARD!

For many of those folks, the overall risks and costs of the procedure seemed to offer little benefit. By 2009, Medicare alone spent $3.5 billion on stents, yet it wasn't always clear that we were getting our money's worth, or that we were placing stents in the right patients, in the right blockages. Dr. Steven Nissen, who at the time was chief of cardiovascular medicine at the prestigious Cleveland Clinic, told the *New York Times* in 2010, "We're spending a fortune as a country on procedures that we don't need."

Part of the reason for that was because we couldn't always "see" very well.

Even Angiograms Have Blind Spots—or at Least They Used To

A seminal 2011 study in the *New England Journal of Medicine* used a technology called "catheter-directed intravascular ultrasound" to see if any atherosclerotic blockages were being missed on a standard angiogram. (In defense of cardiologists, there's a fair amount of art to the science of visually judging the degree of blockage seen on an angiogram.) It turns out that ultrasound "saw" twice as many blockages as the standard angiogram, and compared to ultrasound, an angiogram was far more likely to underestimate the degree of blockage. Over the following three years of the study, about 20% of the patients ended up returning with more problems and getting another angiogram. Half of the time the new problem was due to recurrent disease at the previously treated blockage, and the other half of the time the problem was caused by the growth of a previously noted, but angiographically small (and therefore unstented) blockage.

Fortunately, better technology now allows cardiologists to objectively measure rather than guesstimate the degree of blockage seen on an angiogram. And a newer type of angiogram—a CT coronary angiogram—is changing things too. An angiogram performed in a CT scanner doesn't need a catheter to be threaded up into the heart. Instead it takes a series of rapid images as an intravenous contrast solution moves through the coronary arteries. The 3D images that are subsequently created are very good at detailing plaques, and sometimes find plaques that a conventional (a.k.a. "invasive") angiogram might miss.

A CT coronary angiogram (CTCA) doesn't carry the small yet serious procedural risks that an invasive angiogram does: stroke, heart attack, death, or bleeding. But one downside to a CT angiogram is that it is only diagnostic. If a blockage is found that requires angioplasty, the patient will need an invasive, catheter-guided angiogram to fix it.

CTCAs and other technology like cardiac MRI have allowed physicians to be more discerning about who needs an angiogram. They've taken much of the uncertainty out of the common clinical scenario—"Is this patient's chest pain from coronary artery disease, and if so, do they have a lot or a little?" and they've eliminated a lot of low-yield "let's take a peek, because we'd hate to miss something" angiograms.

Small Plaques Can Sometimes Cause Big Problems

Although conventional and CT coronary angiograms have allowed us to visualize atherosclerotic blockages ("plaques"), they have not given us the ability to look into the future and see which blockages are most likely to cause a heart attack. Historically, it was always the largest plaques that grabbed our attention, and that made sense. But here's where the plumbing metaphor of atherosclerosis sometimes leaves us all wet: with atherosclerosis, *small plaques can sometimes create big problems.*

That's not true in plumbing, where the blockages (excluding sewer rats) and the pipes themselves are inanimate. As I mentioned before, plaques are scars on the inside of a blood vessel wall. They are mechanical but also physiological; they are alive and dynamic, and like a simmering volcano, things can change quickly. They can become unstable and rapidly enlarge (à la Jiffy Pop popcorn) either due to crescendoing inflammation or bleeding into the plaque itself. They can split open, forming a rough spot that attracts a clot that can occlude the entire blood vessel in minutes.

The Problem with Stress Tests: False Assurances Are the Worst Kind of Assurances

The idea that small plaques could cause big problems seemed so counterintuitive that both doctors and patients found relief in what turned out to be false assurances: "You're ok. The angiogram didn't show any big blockages."

It's definitely good news that there weren't any big blockages, but unfortunately that's no guarantee that you're going to be OK. With some regularity a well-known public figure dies suddenly of heart attack caused by a plaque rupture. After a nationally known news anchor died of a cardiac arrest in 2014, his journalist colleagues and the public asked the same question: how could he have died of a heart attack when he'd just had a normal stress test two months earlier?

The answer comes back to the "small can be BIG" paradox. Stress tests can only detect blockages of 70 percent or more; anything less than that and enough blood can squeeze through the gap to make the test normal. Working off a plumbing paradigm, patients like the unfortunate news anchor often got the message "You're in good shape—you've got no evidence of significant coronary disease," when they might well have insignificant coronary disease that could become significant at any moment.

No one was being intentionally misled, but what patients were told, or what they heard, could be misleading. A patient who just had an angioplasty and a stent and was told, "We found a 90 percent blockage and got it down to zero," might forget the part about the smaller stuff that the cardiologist said didn't need to be plumbed. Patients might logically conclude that they *had* coronary artery disease but their doctors got rid of it.

Patients like those go home to a spice rack full of medications and think, "What good are all these pills? And why do I have to keep taking them if the blockage is gone, or if the stress test didn't show any disease?"

The answer has to do with what stents can and cannot do.

What Angioplasty and Stenting Can Do

Stents can save and improve lives. When patients experience a heart attack, the bigger and more serious it is, the more urgently they need angioplasty. For what's termed an "ST-segment-elevation-myocardial infarction" (STEMI), the goal is to have the plugged coronary artery reopened in 90 minutes or less. For those folks, time is muscle:

the quicker the blocked coronary artery can be opened, the less damage to heart, and the better they will do. For patients with a non-STEMI, we've typically got more time, particularly if their symptoms settle down with heart medications and blood thinners.

There are a number of indications for having an angiogram besides having a heart attack—if, for example, one has known coronary disease that is worsening despite optimal medical therapy. The use of angioplasty has also expanded because, as the complexity and capabilities of the procedure has improved, cardiologists are now able to open up complicated blockages that would have previously required bypass surgery.

Medications Lack Razzmatazz, but They Work

What stents cannot do is address the factors that are causing the inflammation and scarring in the first place. Ironically, studies on the efficacy of angioplasty are often presented or viewed as a comparison between those who were randomized to an angioplasty and those who were randomized to be treated "just" with medication. The fact is, *everyone* in the study was being treated with medications, because they work. Remember, if you end up getting a stent, you'll need an additional medication for that too: a blood thinner for a minimum of six months. That can be a real problem if you end up developing a bleeding problem or require some kind of procedure or surgery.

It's true: pills don't offer the razzmatazz and technical wizardry of an angioplasty and stent, but they do work—and better than most of us would guess. Another article in the *New England Journal of Medicine* delved into what factors were involved in the impressive lowering of coronary artery disease deaths in the United States in the 1980s and '90s, when adjusted death rates for such fell by 50 percent.

For all their technical wizardry, blood and gore, open-heart bypass surgery and angioplasty accounted for a mere 7 percent of the gains, and that's because they don't soothe aching arteries. But medications can be very effective at preventing arterial damage by reducing the shearing forces of high blood pressure, preventing blood clots from forming, and calming unstable plaques. Drugs like Lipitor, Zocor, and Crestor don't work like Drano, digesting hairball cholesterol blockages—they work by lowering the levels of "bad cholesterol" (the kind that fuels plaque buildup) and by soothing the inflammation that causes plaques to either grow or rupture.

What to Do

If you already have coronary artery disease, I hope you have a better understanding of what it is (a dynamic process that leads to scarring of the coronary arteries) and what it isn't (purely a plumbing issue). If you have a heart attack, a stent might very well save your life and keep your heart from being seriously injured (leading to heart failure). But not everyone with coronary artery disease needs an angioplasty and a stent, and the best way to avoid getting one (or a second or a third one; or worse yet, open heart surgery) is to address your underlying risk factors.

If you don't have coronary artery disease and would prefer to keep it that way, see the following chapter on heart disease prevention. It will help you get a sense of what your risk of developing cardiovascular disease is, and knowing that, how much effort you might want to devote to avoiding it.

Remember, when it comes to heart disease, prevention beats acute therapy—and if á cardiac arrest is the first warning sign you get, you might not even live long enough to get your emergent angiogram. Follow building codes and hang a smoke detector now so you won't need a fire truck later. Because waiting for a 70 percent blockage to show up on your stress test is a dangerous way to manage the play clock. And waiting for something like an East Siberian brown bear to picnic on your chest might even be considered reckless.

HEART DISEASE PREVENTION

An Ounce of Cardiovascular Disease Prevention Is Worth 453.592 Grams of Cure, in Metric Terms

E veryone will die of something, but come on, there's a limit to how many men can die like J. Howard Marshall, a Texas oil billionaire who, at age 89, famously married Anna Nicole Smith, a buxom 26-year-old model who rose to fame by cornering the silicone market. Marshall died 14 months later of "natural causes."

For the rest of us, a massive heart attack while strapped into a nursing home shower chair could be a mercifully quick and perhaps even welcome Uber ride into the afterlife. But atherosclerotic disease can come much earlier than that, and the results—a weakened heart, or paralysis from a stroke—can be disastrous. Avoiding cardiovascular disease is key to living a longer and more vital life.

Primordial Prevention in Cardiovascular Disease

You've probably heard of primordial stew, the cosmic borscht from which life on Earth crawled out to purportedly exclaim, "Boy, I *hate* the taste of borscht."

MAN OVERBOARD!

To prevent heart disease, treat the causes ("risk factors"): diabetes, high cholesterol and blood pressure, smoking, abdominal obesity, inactivity, stress, and low fruit and vegetable intake. Risk of heart attack or stroke rises sharply with each additional cause. The challenge is to address these risk factors without being consumed by them. Small improvements can bring big benefits.

Well, there's a concept called "primordial prevention," which is the idea that if we can prevent the primary (primordial) trigger in the physiologic chain of disease, then we can shut down the entire process. For example, obesity is the major cause of adult diabetes, which is a major contributor to cardiovascular disease. We can try to prevent the onset of cardiovascular disease by controlling the diabetes, but the best plan would be to prevent the patient from becoming obese in the first place.

The major risk factors for atherosclerosis—the scarring process that causes blood vessels to close off—have been well known, but in 2004, the INTERHEART study looked at more than 15,000 patients in 52 countries who had suffered a heart attack and then calculated which of the known risk factors seemed to be most powerful.

The study found that nine risk factors explained 90 percent of the heart attacks:

- Smoking
- Diabetes
- High blood pressure (hypertension)
- Abdominal obesity
- Elevated cholesterol (dyslipidemia)
- Lack of regular physical activity
- Teetotaling (i.e., no alcohol intake)
- Diet low in fruits and vegetables
- Low psychosocial index (too much depression, work stress, or financial stress)

For any individual man, smoking and bad cholesterol were the strongest factors, each more than tripling the risk of a heart attack. For women, bad cholesterol and strong psychosocial stressors more than tripled their risk, and having diabetes more than quadrupled it. Interestingly, improving healthy lifestyle factors such as eating lots of fruits and vegetables, getting quality exercise, and drinking alcohol moderately were much more beneficial to women than they were to men. (Men, why do we even *try* to be good?)

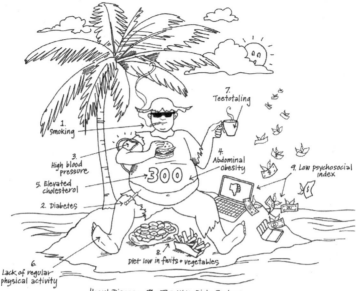

1. Smoking
7. Teetotaling
3. High blood pressure
4. Abdominal obesity
9. Low psychosocial index
5. Elevated cholesterol
2. Diabetes
300
6. Lack of regular physical activity
8. Diet low in fruits + vegetables

Heart Disease: The Top Nine Risk Factors

In an ideal world, the producers of *Survivor* would invite you to participate in their special *Survivor: Nondescript Middle-Aged-Guy* series. Three days later you and your fellow contestants would be dropped off on an Indonesian atoll, where you'd run out of cigarettes in the first six minutes and the dynamic duo of starvation and regular exercise would see your high blood pressure, mildly elevated blood sugars, and 12- to 24-pack abs magically melt away. Wham! You never felt better (except for those nagging nicotine withdrawal symptoms).

On the negative risk factor side, all the sniping and backstabbing on the show would raise your stress levels higher than a coconut tree, which is, coincidentally, where you'd have stashed the home brew you secretly concocted out of fermented jungle roots, smartly recognizing that moderate home brew consumption may be not only heart healthy but also a powerful bargaining chip on a supposedly "dry" atoll.

Future Risks Can Help Guide Present Behavior

Of course, *Survivor* is never going to call you, so let's get back to reality, which is that identifying your risk factors for having a heart attack is a whole lot easier than actually eliminating them. Yes, knowledge can be motivational, but only if it was preceded by ignorance, and is there anything on the INTERHEART risk list that most people didn't already know? Maybe the benefit of moderate alcohol use?

Reminding my patients of what seems obvious—"your liver problems might improve if you stop drinking"—runs the real risk of making them feel stupid or childishly naive. Before COVID-19 began monopolizing health-care headlines, a series of research articles boldly proclaimed that vaping could result in vaping-induced lung injury. No kidding! Who would have ever imagined that inhaling superheated gases into your lungs could lead to lung troubles?

Most of the time, knowing what to do is kind of obvious. Doing it is another matter. Paul the Apostle, of New Testament fame, was likely writing about spiritual rather than health struggles when he wrote the timeless words, "For I have the desire to do what is good, but I cannot carry it out. For I do not do the good I want to do, but the evil I do not want to do—this I keep on doing."

I will leave the motivational speaking to Paul the Apostle, and also Matt Foley, in his van, down by the river (somehow, I think they would have enjoyed each other). But let me point out this caveat of preventive health: preventive measures have the highest payoff for those at the highest risk, and the lowest reward for those at the lowest risk. So it can be enlightening and motivating to figure out what your personal risk of developing cardiovascular disease is.

What Are My Odds?

Understanding that confronting our own mortality is never easy, I'll suggest you go online and find the ASCVD Risk Estimator – American College of Cardiology, www.acc.org. There are several different risk calculators available, each with different nuances, but this one is the most widely recognized.

The data you'll need to enter is pretty straightforward—age, sex, race, smoking history. The only thing that you'll need help on is blood pressure and your cholesterol profile. If you have a number of blood pressure readings or cholesterol numbers, you're probably best off entering the average of those.

After you have entered the information, your 10-year ASCVD (atherosclerotic cardiovascular disease) risk will appear in a blue banner on top of the page. Again, this predicts the likelihood you will experience a heart attack or stroke in the next decade. Yes, you could die from either of those, but DO NOT PANIC AND START TYPING IN CAPITALS FOR MAXIMUM EFFECT: the number you see is not your mortality risk. If there is a lighter banner below your 10-year risk, it reports your optimal ASCVD risk and your lifetime risk. Again, do not panic: this number will seem high, but remember it's a lifetime risk. If you live long enough, developing some cardiovascular disease is almost inevitable; ideally it will come late in life, perhaps when Anna Nicole is preparing you for bed by dousing you in arthritic gel and reading through your stock portfolio for a bedtime story.

Your risk factor percentage will land you in one of four risk categories:

Low (<5 percent)
Borderline (5 percent to 7.4 percent)
Intermediate (7.5 percent to 19.9 percent)
High (>20 percent)

These categories help guide recommendations about what you should do.

How About One of Those Stress Tests, Couldn't That Help?

A stress test is a screening test that has the name recognition of a mammogram and a colonoscopy, but is arguably much more comfortable than having your breasts in a vice or a fiber optic tube up your backside. The classic stress test has the patient walk on a treadmill while the electric activity of the heart is monitored by a cluster of wires taped across the chest. The heart is a combination of muscle and "wires"—tissue that can conduct electricity and stimulate the heart muscle to beat in a coordinated manner.

The electric activity of the heart can be printed out on paper as an electrocardiogram (EKG) or displayed (usually in electro-green) on a bedside monitor that is often used to dramatic effect on medical shows. Even a medical novice can figure out that when the camera pans to the bedside monitor and shows it going from a bumpy *beep...beep...beep* to a flatline *beeeeeeeeeeeeeeep*, things are about to get very tense. The room is going to fill up with some of the best-looking interns Hollywood casting directors could find, and they will reflexively strike model poses as they try to gallantly save the patient's life—or lose it, if the show writers think the patient's story line isn't worth following.

The idea behind a conventional stress test is that if the rising oxygen demands of the exercising heart cannot be met because of a blockage in the coronary arteries, the muscle and electrical tissues of the heart will suffer. This suffering is what we term "ischemia," and it causes the electrical tracing on the monitor to change in predictable ways. A treadmill test can offer other clues as well. A drop in blood pressure during exercise—rather than the increase in blood pressure that should occur normally—is a particularly bad sign.

This "all wired up on a treadmill" approach is the earliest and crudest type of stress test, and has been improved in a number of different ways. Doctors can now use ultrasound to view the squeezing of the heart at rest compared with peak activity. If a portion of the heart doesn't squeeze well during exercise, it's probably because it isn't getting enough blood due to a blockage. In a nuclear stress test, a mildly radioactive tracer is injected into a vein, first at rest, and then again at peak activity. If there is good blood flow, the entire heart should "light up" with the tracer. If part of the heart muscle doesn't take up the tracer, there is likely to be a blockage in the blood flow to that area.

All of these tests are useful, but here's the problem. They can only detect the biggest blockages, the ones that limit blood flow (>70 percent blocked). They cannot detect smaller blockages, which, as I pointed out in the previous chapter, can sometimes suddenly erupt and cause big problems. And besides, if you're trying to prevent coronary artery disease, you'd like to start as early as possible, which means finding the blockages when they are small.

Is a CAC Score Right for You?

As the arterial scarring process progresses, calcium gets deposited. Like graying hair can indicate a maturing body, calcium can be a marker for maturing atherosclerosis, and the amount of calcium buildup can be measured by a coronary artery calcium (CAC) test.

The ASCVD risk factor tools I mentioned earlier try to answer the question, "What is the statistical likelihood of having a heart attack or stroke in the next 10 years?" A CAC test tries to determine if there is actual—not just statistical—evidence of atherosclerosis.

Rather than huffing and puffing on a treadmill while the doctor and a technician have lengthy internal monologues about how paunchy and out of shape you are, for a CAC test, you just lie inside a CT scanner for 10 minutes.

Insurers don't always cover the cost of the test—$100 to $400—which is unfortunate, because it can be a very useful test. In April 2019, the American College of Cardiology and American Heart Association issued updated guidelines recommending CAC testing for those found to be at borderline or intermediate risk by an ASCVD risk factor tool. As a colleague of mine who specializes in heart disease prevention points out, it's the only test we have that trumps age in terms of its ability to predict an individual's cardiovascular death risk.

A CAC test is reported as a "calcium score":

- 1–10 indicates minimal evidence of atherosclerotic plaque buildup, i.e., coronary artery disease (CAD)
- 11–100 mild evidence
- 101–400 moderate evidence
- >400 extensive evidence

Of course, a low score is good news, but it doesn't mean you *couldn't* have CAD; it just means you probably don't have the more advanced kind of blockages that have built up some calcium. And while a high score isn't good news, for technical reasons, it can't tell you whether all that calcium is piled up in one dangerously tight blockage, or spread out evenly within a series of smaller blockages. Only an angiogram can tell you that.

The Earlier the Better: Preventing Heart Disease by Addressing Risk Factors

If you go back to the ASCVD Risk Estimator Plus homepage, there are two additional tabs you can select. The Therapy Impact tab lets you see how specific interventions—starting on a statin cholesterol medication or stopping smoking, for example—could lower your risk. The Advice tab offers specific treatment recommendations for high blood pressure, diabetes, lifestyle changes etc..

Coupling an ASCVD risk factor score with a CAC score can help you decide on how aggressive you might want to be in addressing your risk factors. Assuming you're reading through the *Man Overboard!* chapters in order, you've already read about smoking, obesity and inactivity. So let's finish out the list of the most common cardiovascular risk factors with a quick rundown on diabetes, elevated cholesterol (dyslipidemia), and hypertension.

Diabetes

Diabetes mellitus is a mix of Latin and Greek words meaning "you're going to get sick of checking your blood sugar." Or, if Wikipedia is to be believed—and why not, it's so easy—the name is derived from the words "siphon" and "honey-sweetened." This bears witness to the fact that diabetics lose a lot of extra fluid because all the glucose in their "honey-sweetened" urine sucks ("siphons") extra water out of the kidneys.

This spilling of glucose out into the urine is what explains the classic triad of diabetic symptoms: feeling very thirsty, urinating all the time, and feeling very hungry (the glucose in the urine siphons off calories, too). For those presenting with that triad, blood sugars are typically significantly and obviously elevated, and the diagnosis is clear.

For those who are being screened for diabetes, the most common confirmatory test is called a "hemoglobin A1C test." It measures how much glucose is stuck to hemoglobin—the molecule in red blood cells that binds oxygen. It gives us a sense of what a person's blood glucose levels have been like for the last several months; the higher the blood sugar, the more glucose there is to bind to hemoglobin, the higher the A1C.

You don't have to be Dr. Oz to know that diabetes has something to do with elevated blood sugars and insulin. With that in mind, there are two types of diabetes:

- Type 1 typically starts in childhood or as a young adult. The cells in the pancreas that make insulin get wiped out, and since there is no insulin to escort glucose out of the blood and into cells, blood sugars rise.
- Type 2 diabetes is often referred to as "adult-onset diabetes." But because it is closely linked to abdominal obesity, and since people are becoming fatter, sooner, even kids can develop this type of diabetes. Whereas type 1 diabetics have little to no insulin, type 2 diabetics typically have high levels of insulin and high levels of insulin resistance. That's because fat makes insulin much less effective, so the pancreas needs to produce higher amounts of insulin to move glucose out of the bloodstream and into the tissues where it is needed.

Type 1 diabetics need to use insulin, but type 2 diabetics can typically be treated with a variety of medications that lower blood glucose levels in different ways. If type 2 diabetes goes on too long, the pancreas can burn out and stop making insulin. Then that patient will need to be on insulin, too. Weight loss can often cure type 2 diabetes if it's not too far advanced, and even moderate weight loss can dramatically improve its control.

Controlling blood sugars is the focus of treating type 2 diabetes, but it's not clear that high blood glucose explains the entire physiologic picture. Tight control of a diabetic's blood sugars improves many of the hallmark injuries of the disease—damage to the eyes, kidneys, nerves—but even tightly controlled diabetics are still at increased risk for cardiovascular disease. In other words, we can normalize your blood sugars, but your physiology is still not normal and we can't do much about that part of the equation, particularly as long as obesity is an issue. That might be changing, as several new classes of diabetic drugs—SGLT2 inhibitors and GLP-1 agonists—not only improve blood sugar control, but also have *proven* cardiovascular benefits. Their novelty and cost makes them what we diplomatically call "spendy," which is also why these new diabetic medications seem to be sponsoring most of daytime television.

Of note, efforts at tight control can create "overshoot" low blood sugar (hypoglycemia) events, and there is increasing awareness that these hypoglycemic events take a toll on brain function. Finding a healthy balance between high and low blood sugar is essential.

Dyslipidemia (Bad Cholesterol)

Dyslipidemia is medicalese for what may be better known as "bad cholesterol." Several decades ago, researchers began to see an association between high cholesterol, saturated fat intake, and atherosclerotic disease. Cholesterol became a four-letter word, *even poisonous*, so for a while, eating an egg for breakfast was considered a suicide attempt. You might as well roll it up in bacon and smoke it. In our darkest hour, we were even frying up things called "egg substitutes."

We often think of fat and cholesterol as being the unwanted detritus of our calorically rich society, but both are critical to our bodily function. Fats, both saturated and unsaturated, are attached to a molecule of glycerol to form triglycerides (you've heard of those). Triglycerides are an important fuel source for the body. The liver manufactures them from carbohydrates (preferably) or protein. If we latch onto more calories than we need, triglycerides can be stored in fat cells, and if you have more of those than you need, you can ask a plastic surgeon to freeze, suck, burn, or laser fry them out of there, aka liposuction.

Cholesterol's principal function, along with a group of chemicals called "phospholipids," is to be the building block of cell membranes. Without membranes it would just be acellular anarchy, our bodies lying there in a pool of salty water, like Frosty the Snowman when he got locked in the greenhouse by the wickedly sadistic magician, till he came to life one day.

Cholesterol is also the main ingredient in bile salts, which come from the liver and are important in absorbing fat from our diet. And it's also the basic chemical structure for numerous hormones in the body. These hormones include not only a number of unheralded maintenance hormones secreted by the adrenal glands, but also limelight sex hormones like progesterone, estrogen, and testosterone.

The liver is the middleman in the story of fat and cholesterol. It packages cholesterol, phospholipids, and triglycerides into little globules called "lipoprotein." The proteins in lipoproteins help the fatty lipids stay dissolved in the watery blood, and they help direct how and where the various components of each package are off-loaded to tissues and organs throughout the body.

You may think you've never heard of lipoproteins, but you probably have—at least, if you've ever had your cholesterol checked. Besides total cholesterol, the test typically includes LDLs (low-density lipoproteins), HDLs (high-density lipoproteins), and triglycerides.

LDL is the lipoprotein in which almost all of the triglycerides have been removed, leaving an especially high concentration of cholesterol and a moderate concentration of phospholipids. It's the high cholesterol part that's the trouble. When the inner lining of a blood vessel, the intima, is damaged—by cigarette smoking, for example—the injury attracts LDLs and also a certain kind of white blood cell called a "monocyte." As the LDL and monocytes move into the intima, the monocytes start engulfing the cholesterol-rich LDLs, releasing chemicals that cause inflammation and further damage. As the damage progresses, a tiny scar becomes a much larger atherosclerotic plaque—the hallmark of atherosclerotic disease.

This is why LDLs are referred to as "bad cholesterol." By comparison, HDL is Glinda the Good. HDLs have high concentrations of protein and small amounts of cholesterol and phospholipids. They seem to be able to prevent, or at least mitigate, the damage done by LDLs. Although low HDL levels carry an *increased* risk of coronary artery disease, we've had a hard time showing that raising their levels actually improves cardiovascular risk.

The question is how to lower your cholesterol (and therefore LDL) levels. Avoiding excessive dietary cholesterol can help, but serum (or total) cholesterol doesn't budge all that much—perhaps 15 to 20 percent—with cholesterol-ducking dietary changes. That's because of a feedback loop with the liver: if you stop eating cholesterol, the liver will eventually notice and begin gearing up and making more. How much more, and to what level, probably is dependent on your familial/genetic profile. Remember, you need *some* cholesterol to live. Vegans, and *Survivor* contestants who are eating their fingernail shavings and the casings off the television production power cables, *still* have cholesterol levels.

So yes, it's helpful to limit dietary cholesterol, but it might make more sense to focus on 1) avoiding saturated fat (typically from animal fat) because it increases cholesterol by 15 percent to 25 percent; and 2) embracing a diet high in unsaturated fats (typically from plant oils), which have a cholesterol-lowering effect.

Dietary changes do work, but they require some effort, and sometimes the cholesterol set point of the liver you inherited from your parents is higher than we'd like. In that case, the next step is to start a statin, a class of drugs that has become widely known for its success in fighting and preventing atherosclerotic disease—and also because massive marketing campaigns have made them household names: Lipitor, Zocor, Crestor. Statins inhibit the ability of the liver to make cholesterol, and LDL levels can fall by 25 percent to 50 percent. That's a big deal because according to the 2018 American Heart Association/American College of Cardiology cholesterol guidelines, each 1% drop in LDL lowers one's cardiovascular risk by roughly 1%. The effect is stronger for those starting out with very high LDLs, but the benefits continue even at lower LDL levels, affirming the general principle that for LDLs, "lower is better."

Although the benefit of statins is thought to be primarily related to this sharp drop in LDL, they also have a soothing effect on the inflammation that stirs the simmering atherosclerotic plaque. We don't understand this process well, but a testament to this idea is the fact that other drugs that have improved patients' LDL and HDL levels didn't similarly reduce atherosclerotic disease events. So the statins have a certain feng shui, and if you have documented atherosclerosis you should probably be taking one, even if your cholesterol level is fantabulous.

Statins raise HDLs and lower triglycerides. So do exercise, weight loss, and lowering saturated fat intake. We have medications other than statins that will lower triglycerides, as will omega-3 fish oils, but neither has been shown to lower the risk of stroke or heart attack very much, if at all. So what's a healthy cholesterol level? An LDL less than 100 mg/dL and an HDL higher than 40 mg/dL. In a perfect world, and particularly if one has already developed coronary artery disease, an LDL of less than 70 is the goal.

Hypertension

According to the CDC, 116 million Americans—nearly half of all adults—have hypertension, or high blood pressure. It's also been labeled a "silent killer," which it gives it an air of intrigue, a spooky feeling. It's more like the wind—measurable but unseen—except you can feel the wind. Hypertension has no symptoms, hence the "silent" descriptor. On rare occasions patients can have a hypertensive crisis, where their blood pressure hits the roof and they develop chest pain, blurred vision, or headache. But the rest of the 116 million Americans with hypertension don't feel a thing, and if they never get a blood pressure cuff wrapped around their biceps (the brachial artery to be more specific), they will remain undiagnosed. Life will be good until the constant pounding on the blood vessels causes a stroke, or kidney or heart failure.

And by the way, there's no "hyper" in hypertension, in the sense that this is not a disease confined to hyperactive type-A personalities. Fuhged-daboudit. When betting on the blood pressure of the highly strung versus the laid back, flip a coin. And then get yourself a blood pressure cuff.

Who Is and Who Ain't in the World of Hypertension? Nearly Half of the Population Might Have It, but Which Half?

You'd like to think that a blood pressure cuff will settle the highly strung vs. laid back wager, but it's not that easy. Blood pressure readings naturally fluctuate—that's healthy, that's physiological. If you're chasing your misbehaving couch-gouging cat around the house with a squirt bottle, your blood pressure *should* go up. When we perform a stress test on a patient, one indicator of fitness and heart health is how high they can get their blood pressure and pulse, and then how quickly it normalizes after exercise (the faster the better).

And although it's absolutely true that high blood pressure leads to strokes and heart attacks, it's a slow process. It doesn't occur from a couple of elevated readings, but rather from months and often years of hypertension.

Sure, you hear stories about someone who got in a car accident, after which their blood pressure shot up, and then they had a stroke; but that scenario typically involves a bursting blood vessel in the brain that ruptures under the transiently high pressure. That's not how the majority of strokes occur. A few elevated blood pressure readings are no cause for panic, just attention.

So the diagnostic question isn't whether you've ever had an elevated blood pressure reading, but rather whether you're consistently hypertensive. For obvious reasons, an occasional blood pressure reading on your annual clinic physical, or a trip to the local pharmacy, doesn't provide a lot of data points. What can provide more data, and more real-life data, is something called "ambulatory blood pressure monitoring" (ABPM)— "ambulatory" as in walking, not as in paramedics with lights blazing. Patients are fitted with a blood pressure cuff that inflates every 20 minutes or so for a 24-hour period, no matter where you are or what you're doing, even while you sleep. It records the data, which your doctor can then download and assess.

For multiple reasons, ambulatory blood pressure monitoring is considered the gold standard for diagnosing hypertension. In fact, the National Health Service in the UK now recommends that every new diagnosis of hypertension be confirmed with ABPM prior to starting medication. For a variety of reasons, ABPM has been slow to catch on here in the United States. It used to be an expensive test, but microprocessors and the computer revolution (you may have heard of it?) have made the technology more accurate and more affordable than ever before, and ABPM has shown us what we're missing:

- **White coat hypertension:** About 20 percent of patients who are consistently hypertensive in the clinic don't have high blood pressure the rest of the day.

- **Masked hypertension:** This is the yin to the yang of white coat hypertension, wherein office blood pressures are normal, but readings outside of the clinic are high. Perhaps "white coat normal-tension" might be a better name for this phenomenon, but it appears that 10 percent of those with normal office blood pressures are being stalked by the silent killer the rest of the day. They just don't know it.
- **Resistant hypertension:** Some people's blood pressure requires multiple medications and still won't come under control. It's resistant to aggressive treatment. One-fifth of those who seem to have stubbornly resistant hypertension are actually well controlled or even *overcontrolled* by out-of-office numbers. They don't need more medication, and they may even need less.
- **Non-dippers:** Most healthy individuals are what are called "dippers." An hour or so into sleep, our blood pressure should fall by 10 percent to 20 percent and then stay low until shortly before awakening. But some people turn out to be non-dippers, showing no drop in their sleeping blood pressure. Studies show that non-dippers are at the highest risk of any hypertensive patient to develop organ damage such as heart failure or kidney disease, so finding and treating them might bring the biggest bang for our pharmaceutical buck.

As you can see, random blood pressure readings with a standard cuff aren't a serious answer to what is a serious and widespread disease. They leave too many people undiagnosed and untreated, and treat too many people who either don't need treatment, or don't need as much medication as they're prescribed. If ambulatory blood pressure monitoring is not available to you, the next best thing would be to buy or borrow a quality home blood pressure monitor, take several good readings a day for a couple of weeks, and then average them. More data, and better data, means better treatment.

What constitutes high blood pressure (HBP)? Here are the numbers:

Normal: less than 120/80
Elevated: 120–129/80

HBP Stage 1: 130–139/80–89
HBP Stage 2: 140+/90+
HBP Crisis: >180/120

Treatment generally starts at HBP Stage 1 for anyone with established cerebrovascular disease, or significant risk factors for such; or at HBP Stage 2 for those at low risk. Your physician will help you figure it out.

Addressing Your Risk Factors Without Being Consumed by Them

Depending on your cardiovascular risk and your personality type, managing your risk factors can potentially get very complicated. You can tie yourself up in knots, like the famous "square Turk's head knot," or the elusive "bowline on a bight knot." I have seen this happen. It's terrible. So here are a few things to keep in mind.

Overall Risk Rises Sharply with Increasing Number of Risk Factors

Let's enter some hypothetical numbers into the ACC ASCVD Risk Estimator Plus tool and see what happens. A 57-year-old male author with good blood pressure and cholesterol, and with no smoking, diabetes, or medications registers a 10-year ASCVD risk score of 4 %. The author goes on a whirlwind multi-state book tour and gains an enormous amount of weight grazing at truck stops off the interstate. The extra weight gives him Stage 2 high blood pressure; he starts on medication, and his ASCVD risk score rises to 7%. The anxiety of being on blood pressure pills (and also, frankly, stalled book sales) causes him to eat even more, and further weight gain gives him diabetes, pushing his ASCVD risk score to 13%. In a desperate and ill-fated attempt to curtail his appetite and weight gain, he begins smoking, which cranks his ASCVD risk up to 22%.

The lesson here: avoid whirlwind book tours and truck stop buffets—and also, notice that increasing risk factors can cause overall risk to rise sharply. One risk factor caused the baseline risk to increase by 70%, adding a second increased it by 3-fold, and adding a third by 5-fold. The good news is that the reverse is also true: the overall risk numbers can fall just as precipitously when individual risk factors are either removed (smoking) or improved (HBP, cholesterol, diabetes).

The Higher the Risk, the Higher the Benefit from Treatment, and Vice Versa—the Lower the Risk, the Less That Treatment Has to Offer You

Which seems more satisfying and productive: sweeping up a dirty floor, or an almost clean floor? The dirty one of course: the results are more dramatic and justify our efforts. In the same vein, the lower your absolute risk of developing a particular disease, the less benefit any treatment or preventative intervention—even the finest in the land—can offer you. Hypertension is a symptomless disease, so you don't treat it to feel better; you treat it to lower your risk of cardiovascular disease. If your risk is otherwise low, the benefit of taking blood pressure medication will be lower, too. There will still be a benefit, but it's not worth the mortal fixation that some people have with their medication, as if a missed pill or an isolated elevated blood pressure reading is akin to signing your own death certificate.

This nuanced but honest message is not always conveyed very well in public health messaging, which tends to be emphatic and absolute, more like the God in Hebrew scriptures, a lot of smiting and smoting: "Eat thy spinach, or thou shalt die, and when thou art are on thy death bed, thou shalt *crave* spinach, and no one—nay, not one—will press it to thy lips." Doctors are guilty of this infraction: we sometimes scare people to death as we try to scare them to health.

Take aspirin, for example. Take one right now, because "an aspirin a day keeps the doctor away," right? That's what we've been telling many patients for years. And while that is true on a public health level—aspirin can prevent strokes and heart attacks in a large population of people—for individual patients at low risk, the benefits of a daily aspirin are very small. Unfortunately the risks of side effects, primarily stomach ulcers and gastrointestinal bleeding, stay the same, regardless of the individual's stroke risk. For someone at low risk, an aspirin a day is more likely *not* to keep the doctor away; in fact, they might want to *find* a doctor so they can talk about the blood in their stool.

Our strongest recommendations often come from our most powerful studies—randomized, controlled trials—but even those have results that can be misleading. The headline might read FERMENTED JUNGLE ROOT MOONSHINE LOWERS STROKE RISK BY 20%, but that doesn't mean that everyone in the study benefited; much of that benefit may have gone to the small minority of trial participants who were at the highest risk. Many imbibers may have had no benefit at all. Some may have drunk the moonshine and doggie-paddled off into the ocean at night, never to be seen again. Some may have fallen out of the coconut tree and injured themselves.

The better you understand your risk of any particular disease, the better you'll be able to assess the benefits and risks of any treatment.

More Might Be Better, but How Much Better? And at What Cost?

When it comes to treating blood pressure and elevated cholesterol, the biggest bang for the buck comes at moderate doses. It's the law of diminishing returns: you pay big bucks to complete the last 5 percent of a job. There's a lot of emphasis now on what's called "targeted therapy," where patients are encouraged to get their blood pressure or cholesterol to a target number. And doctors are increasingly being graded on whether or not they get patients to that target.

For example, there's definitely some additional benefit in getting your LDL to less than 70 if you've had a previous heart attack. But if you brought it down from 135 to 78 with diet, exercise, and a low-dose statin, maxing out your statin dose or adding another drug may not be worth the small, fractional risk reduction you'd get by driving the LDL to below 70. "More" is sometimes too much.

What's the goal? To maximize your health and enjoy your life, not to obsess about your last cholesterol check, your last blood pressure, or your last HbA1C (a measure of diabetic control). Aggressive risk factor reduction can have real payoffs, but take it easy on yourself: life shouldn't be the death of you.

17 CANCER, THE BIG "C"

Nixon Declared War on Cancer; Cancer Missed the Memo

E veryone dies of something, and for a few unsuspecting folks, the end will come from… an asteroid. Wouldn't that be exciting?

A report from the National Research Council calculated that over a millennia or so, an average of 91 people a year will be killed by high-and-tight interplanetary beanballs. The fact that we have a hard time drumming up the name of *anyone* in modernity killed by an asteroid (although a cow was killed in Venezuela in 1972) suggests that, statistically speaking, we're in a significant death-by-asteroid lull. Don't look up.

Rather than looking to the heavens to contemplate death by asteroid, which would save you a pile of money on cremation services, why not focus on a more likely end-of-life scenario?

Cancer and heart disease jockey back and forth for position as the leading cause of death of US men after age 45. Prostate cancer (not *prostrate* cancer, which is exceedingly rare—it hits you only when you're lying down) is the most

MAN OVERBOARD!

Prostate cancer most common, followed by lung and colon. Lung most lethal. Most cancers grow locally, then move into lymph nodes, then franchise (metastasize) themselves to other organs. Lung cancer is like a bad house guest: shows up late, drunk, and hostile. Chance of cure best if able to surgically remove. Colon cancer is more forgiving—easier to find early via colonoscopy, and more easily treated. Prostate cancer is an odd bugger. The question isn't exactly who will get it (a majority of men will, if they live long enough), but what kind: the aggressive kind, or the docile, slow-growing, microscopic kind whose only symptom is a mildly elevated PSA?

common cancer in men. Lung cancer is the second most common cancer in men, and colorectal cancer is third.

Although prostate, lung, and colon cancers are the most frequently *diagnosed* cancers in men, lung cancer is the deadliest of the three by a couple of furlongs. For women, substitute breast cancer for prostate cancer and the two lists—most common and most deadly—are the same.

As I mentioned in the prologue, nearly all health disparities observed between races are not due to the construct (or concept) we call "race," but are rather due to cultural differences (diet being a common factor) or social determinants of health such as poverty, physical and financial barriers to accessing health care and healthy food, etc. With that disclaimer in mind, there are some wrinkles in the racial demographics of cancer that are worth noting.

Grouping all races together, the most commonly diagnosed male cancers in order are prostate, lung, and colon. That order holds for Whites, Asians and Pacific Islanders, and Blacks, although among Blacks, prostate cancer is particularly common—more than lung and colon cancer combined. For Hispanics, colon moves ahead of lung cancer—the order being prostate, colon, lung.

Looking at the most common cause of cancer *deaths* for all races together, the order is lung, prostate, colon, with lung cancer being particularly common—more than prostate and colon cancer combined. That order holds for Whites, Hispanics, and Blacks, although for Blacks, the number of deaths from prostate cancer is much closer to

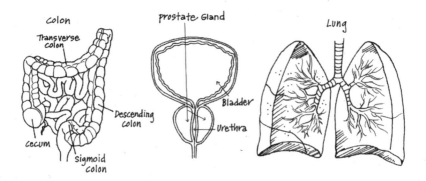

MAN OVERBOARD!

that of lung cancer. For Asians and Pacific Islanders, the order is lung, liver, colon, and then prostate.

There's a little bit of homework to do before we take a closer look at this trifecta of male cancers. Let's start with the obvious question:

What, Exactly, Is Cancer?

If you want an encyclopedic read on the history of cancer, you should pick up the Pulitzer Prize–winning book *The Emperor of All Maladies*. However, if you're a slow reader, there's a decent chance that you will develop cancer by the time you finish the book. It's that long. I would recommend it though—the book, that is, not cancer.

Here's a truncated explanation: cancer is out-of-control cell growth.

Throughout our lives, our bodies are in a state of perpetual renewal. Old cells wear out, die off, and are replaced by new ones. You cut yourself shaving, and new cells need to grow to heal the wound—in moderation. Too many cells, and too much growth, and you'll end up with a fin of tissue growing off the edge of your jaw that makes you look like a character from *Star Trek: The Next Generation*.

At the beginning of human life, once the egg completes a successful merger with the sperm and all the papers are signed and notarized, growth is the dominant theme until we reach adulthood. Thereafter we move into a maintenance phase, a steady state, where the number of new cells being created equals those that are wearing out and being recycled.

It is both elegant and miraculous. If the human body were a house, that house would be perpetually remodeling itself, replacing aging timbers, drywall, tiles, electrical wires, paint, and plumbing with new stuff. (This perpetual body remodel is entirely different from the home remodel concepts of a partner who is always dreaming of something new and costly.)

Cancer begins when a single cell goes rogue. If life is an infinitely large and complex orchestra, cancer is the saxophone player abandoning both the conductor and the musical score. Mutations in DNA (the blueprints for how a cell behaves) cause the cell to begin dividing rapidly all on its own, ignoring a complex array of signals that are designed to keep growth in check.

It is not typically one single mutation (genetic error) that transforms a normal cell into a cancerous one, but mutations beget mutations, and they pile up. It is common for breast and colon cancer cells to have 50 to 80 gene mutations. It is a smaller number of those mutations—perhaps as few as 10—that directly contribute to the cancerous behavior of the cells. The rest of the mutations are more likely "bystander" errors: mutations that occurred as part of the fast and sloppy cell replication inherent to all malignancies.

How can a single rogue line of cells take down its much larger host? Back when tuberculosis was common and untreatable, its victims were said to have died of consumption. This description fits cancer to a tee. Yes, some cancers can be in a particularly bad spot, compressing the brain or blocking a bile duct, but most overpower their hosts by consumption. The rapidly dividing, high-metabolic-rate cancer cells quite literally suck the energy and resources out of the body. They also secrete a host of poorly understood but wildly abnormal chemicals that poison the rest of the body, squelching one's appetite, sapping energy, and making the blood stickier and more prone to clotting.

The sax player clones herself, then plays louder and faster until the orchestra is too confused and exhausted to keep up. And besides, no one can hear them anymore.

Every Form of Cancer Is Unique, but the Initial Approach Is the Same

Each kind of cancer—thyroid cancer, leukemia, melanoma—has its own unique profile in terms of how fast it grows, its ability to spread to other organs, how easy is it to detect, and what kind of treatments it requires.

But there are also some commonalities across the spectrum that provide a framework for understanding how we diagnose and treat cancer.

First, the diagnosis must be confirmed. That typically means putting a needle into the suspect area and removing a plug of tissue—a biopsy. That sample is then examined by a pathologist—a lab-based doctor who uses complicated lab tests and microscopes rather than a stethoscope or a CT scan to do his or her work.

The pathologist makes the call on whether a biopsy is cancerous, including what kind of cancer it is, how cancerous it appears to be (cells that are more malignant appear more gnarly and twisted under a microscope) and if there is any evidence that the cancer has spread outside of the organ that it started in.

Cancer can spread directly, like in the movie *The Blob*, engulfing everything in its path except the lead actor, Steve McQueen. Or it can move into the lymphatic system that drains that particular organ. Lymph channels are the back alleyways of the body, a slow-flow pathway that drains away waste products and extra fluid and returns them, eventually, to the bloodstream. Scattered along these lymph channels are bean-shaped lymph nodes—enclaves of white blood cells that help cleanse the lymph fluid, removing debris and killing off viruses, bacteria, or cancerous cells (if we're lucky).

If cancer thumbs a ride via an artery or a vein, it can end up settling down in a distant organ. For instance, a melanoma on the leg can end up in the brain. We call this "metastatic disease," and it is important for two reasons.

First, when a cancer metastasizes to another organ, it retains the unique and particular features and behaviors of its organ of origin. In other words, prostate cancer that spreads to the bones still behaves like prostate cancer. Lung cancer that has spread to the brain still responds to lung cancer treatments, and not to brain cancer therapies. This "organ of origin" concept also dictates how we talk about cancer. Prostate cancer that has spread to the bones would not be called "bone cancer," but rather "prostate cancer with bone metastases." Lung cancer that has spread to the brain would not be termed "brain cancer," but rather "lung cancer with brain metastases." If cancer appears in multiple places at once, the pathologist looking at the biopsy will usually be able to tell us what organ the cancer originated in.

Second, metastatic cancer typically suggests a more aggressive, more advanced form of cancer that will be difficult to cure (although there are a few exceptions like lymphoma or testicular cancer).

In cases where it makes sense to surgically remove the cancer, the pathologist will look at what was extracted in the operating room to see whether cancer cells have grown outside of the organ and into the lymph nodes. Besides examining these microscopic clues, CT, MRI, or PET scanning are commonly used to look for evidence of cancer spread. PET scans use a radioactive tracer to identify tissues anywhere in the body that have high metabolic activity—a strong indicator for cancer.

All this is part of what's called "cancer staging." Putting cancers into different stages based on their appearance and spread has allowed us to refine which treatments work best for each particular stage of that cancer.

There's Never Been a Better Time to Get Cancer

I'm joking, but I am not joking. Of course there never has been, and never will be, a good time to have cancer. But if one does, there's never been a better time to get cancer treatment. That's because we're in the midst of an incredible revolution in how and how well we treat cancer, a revolution that brings us back to the desk of the pathologist.

Think of how criminal prosecution has changed in recent years. Witness testimony—often flawed or biased and always unscientific—has been replaced by video footage, cell phone tracking data, and DNA analysis that can definitively identify the perpetrator. A case that went cold 20 years ago can be solved with a swab of cells off someone's cheek.

Similarly, pathologists now have an ever-expanding toolbox of genetic and biomolecular tests that are rapidly making yesterday's cancer therapy look like Homer Simpson in the role of Sherlock Holmes—bungling, antiquated, dangerous even (but not for the criminals).

Cancer genomics is the ability to identify the specific mutations in the DNA of any specific cancer. This information is being entered into a national database, the Cancer Genome Atlas, and will provide us with much better information about the particular kind of cancer each patient has—its aggressiveness, its ability to metastasize.

As we will discuss later, prostate cancer is most commonly a slow-growing disease that smolders for years or even decades prior to becoming clinically apparent. And yet, on some occasions, it shows up in a fast-and-furious mode in a middle-aged man. Genomic analysis might help us figure out why. An oncologist might say, "This tumor has five of seven mutations needed to become resistant to our treatment, and it has two of the three mutations needed to metastasize out of the prostate. This one needs to be treated and watched closely."

Novel Therapies: The End of Carpet-Bombing

The toll that cancer treatment takes on cancer patients is well known. Up until recently, cancer treatment included three major options:

- Surgery (cut it out)
- Chemotherapy (poison it)
- Radiation (burn it up)

Over time, these treatments have become more refined, but hardly perfected.

Surgery has its operative risks and recovery issues, and because we still cannot see microscopic amounts of cancer on CT scans and MRIs, sometimes surgery doesn't end up being the cure we hoped it would be. The surgeon thought she got it all out (the pathologist confirmed this on the analysis of the surgically removed specimen). But microscopic amounts of cancerous cells—too small to be detected by staging CT or MRI scans—were still left behind. Eventually the cancer grows back, either at the surgical site (local recurrence) or somewhere else, as metastatic disease.

Radiation and chemotherapy work in different ways, but the idea is to kill cancer cells while leaving healthy cells alone. Although both treatments have been exponentially refined and improved over the years, they still have significant toxicities and side effects—collateral damage in the war on cancer. People getting these treatments can sometimes feel like they've been poisoned because, well, they have been (for what we hope will be a good cause).

Enter two novel treatment modalities called "targeted therapy" and "immunotherapy."

Targeted therapies look for proteins that are very specific to the cancer cells. Researchers then design molecules that can bind to those proteins. Targeted therapies work in different ways depending on what specific protein is being targeted, but the goal is the same: stopping the growth and spread of cancer.

Prior to the discovery of the first targeted therapy (imatinib mesylate/Gleevec), the diagnosis of chronic myelogenous leukemia (CML) was fatal. Now, for most CML patients, Gleevec can keep their CML subdued and in remission for years, or perhaps a lifetime. The cancerous cells are still there, hanging around in small numbers, but the patient feels healthy. Like taking insulin to control diabetes, the formerly fatal CML has become a chronic illness than can be controlled with medication.

Immunotherapy works by helping our immune system find and remove cancerous cells. The immune system's job description includes eliminating viruses, bacteria, and other would-be invaders, but it also includes the removal of cancerous cells. Sometimes cancer cells acquire the ability to evade our immune system, allowing them to grow and spread incognito. As with targeted therapies, different immunotherapies work in different ways. One well-known immunotherapy is pembrolizumab (Keytruda). It binds to a protein called PD-1, thereby blocking the tumor's ability to inactivate the immune cell. "Gotcha! I've inactivated your inactivator!"

Cancer Screening Basics
Looking for Trouble and Hoping Not to Find It

Screening for cancer reminds me of organizing a family reunion. The idea itself is an excellent one, so well intentioned and full of hope. After all, blood is thicker than water, and these are the ties that bind. We'll tie a tire swing to the family tree and tell stories!

And yet the thing itself ends up being far more complicated. Sometimes the blood that flows down through the ages seems to clot, and then it stops flowing; sometimes the ties that bind give people rope burns, or worse yet, PTSD. Some people get nauseated on a nostalgic tire swing.

Sometimes cancer screening is less effective and more complicated than we had hoped. In a perfect world, cancer screening would work like a smoke alarm. The fire is detected early and is easily extinguished. Of course, there can be false alarms—the cheese slips off the pizza and the oven is belching smoke but is not on fire—but these are easily managed. Smoke detectors are designed with such finesse and sensitivity that they won't sleep through a fire. They always work.

Cancer screenings are a lot clumsier than smoke detectors. They miss some cancers, mostly because all cancers begin microscopically and we still don't see well at that level. Sometimes these tests call things "cancer" that aren't—they are false alarms that typically mean additional testing and a lot of worry, not just hitting the reset button on a smoke alarm.

Even when screening tests work perfectly and find cancer in its earliest stages, you still have to have a treatment option that allows you to capitalize on the early warning. If I tied you to a goalpost, gave you a short-range weapon like a .22 caliber pistol, and then released a hungry grizzly bear from the other end zone, handing you a good set of binoculars wouldn't really change the outcome. The last 10 yards would still tell the tale; the other 90 yards would just give you more time to stare at your nemesis and fill your shorts—which, yes, depending on volume, odor, and prevailing winds, could be a deterrent.

There's a name for this phenomenon: lead time bias. Let's say that there's a terrible cancer called "stuffed green peppers cancer" that, even with the most aggressive treatment and a whole lot of ketchup, kills everyone within five years of the diagnosis. Then a screening test is invented that detects the dreaded stuffed green peppers cancer an average of three years earlier. On the face of it, screening appears to have improved the survival to eight years, when in reality, the test added three years of the grief that can come with living with a diagnosis of cancer but didn't change the end point—the actual outcome.

In the last decade or so, the trend in screening guidelines has been toward recommending less frequent, and fewer, routine cancer screenings.

These recommendations [for less routine screening] are based on an evolving—if counterintuitive—understanding that more screening does not necessarily translate into fewer cancer deaths and that some screening may actually do more harm than good.
—National Cancer Institute, National Institutes of Health

Cancer Prevention

Like Cavities and Telemarketers, It's Best to Avoid Cancer in the First Place

President Richard Nixon declared war on cancer back in the 1970s, but apparently cancer never got the message. It remains in a virtual tie with cardiovascular disease as the leading cause of death, and might well have taken sole possession of first place if we hadn't gone on an obesity bender that gave heart disease "new life," so to speak.

In a war where cancer is the enemy, forget what they say about bravery and courage: sometimes running away as fast as you can is a very legitimate military maneuver.

If you want to skip out on all the life lessons that getting cancer can give you, the top 10 things on the list should be to *avoid smoking*, because both first- and secondhand smoke increase the risk of getting every imaginable malignancy except the Tropic of Cancer. And chewing tobacco (pronounced "tuh-BACK-er" in the language of the ancient Duck Dynasty) teams up with alcohol to be major risk factors for developing oral cancer (you can literally "save face"—and tongue and jaw and throat—by ditching the dip or the chaw).

If you are a smoker, *do not move on to other avoidance areas* until you have successfully completed the Vices chapter and memorized the Smoker's Amalgamated Sinners' and Serenity Prayer. The stuff is *that bad*. In the disease-prevention version of Monopoly, smoking cessation is Board-walk with a hotel—the big payday—and everything else is Baltic Avenue occupied by your mother-in-law's nearly defunct scrapbooking store.

Here are some numbers to consider. Smoking caused the premature death of 100 million people in the 20th century, and it's shooting to send 1 billion people to an early shower in the 21st century. Sucking on the heaters shortens a smoker's life by an average of a decade, and it lowers the chance of ever becoming an octogenarian by 30 percent.

But the good news is that the body can forgive. If you quit before age 35, you'll carry on with your life with no additional excess risk of death. Past age 35, saddling up and riding your way out of Marlboro country can still dramatically reduce—but not eliminate—the excess risk of death smoking stowed away in your saddlebags. So cut it out, the sooner the better.

Once you've plucked the lowest-hanging and juiciest carcinogenic fruit (cigarettes), you can climb the ladder (careful!) to reach some of the higher-hanging cancer risk factors.

Sun Exposure

You can avoid skin cancer by limiting your cumulative sun exposure (the trigger for typically milder forms of skin cancer such as basal cell and squamous cell) and by avoiding sunburns (the trigger for the more lethal melanoma).

Radon in the Basement Man Cave

You can have your basement tested for radon (the second leading cause of lung cancer). Lung cancer is rising in nonsmokers, and the increase is very likely due to a long list of environmental toxins we inhale. If you don't live next to a volcanic vent, which can release all kinds of toxic gases, then radon is the likely culprit. It's an invisible, odorless gas that's literally everywhere, but at low levels. It's the high levels we worry about, and those are typically found in the basement. Get it checked.

Human Papilloma Virus Vaccine Prevents Cancer

Human papilloma virus (HPV) causes more than 90% of cervical cancer. So when an HPV vaccine came out in 2006, it seemed that the benefit was primarily for women. The thinking was, since HPV is spread by sexual activity, young boys should also be vaccinated to prevent spreading the virus to female partners. Over time though, the list of cancers caused by HPV has grown to include penile cancer, anal cancer, and cancer of the back of the tongue and tonsils. It's estimated that vaccination could prevent more than 90% of all HPV cancers, but vaccination works best if given before sexual activity begins. That's why vaccination is recommended for all adolescents age 11 or 12, and is not recommended for adults older than 26, where the benefit is felt to be low.

Booze Blues

Regular, heavier alcohol intake increases the risk of colon cancer, and together with smoking is the major cause of mouth and throat cancers.

Eat Your Fruits and Vegetables, but Skip the Supplements

We know that people who have a diet rich in fruits and vegetables have a lower incidence of cancer, but to date, no study has shown that taking vitamin supplements will lower your risk of cancer. Fruits and vegetables are indeed rich in vitamins and minerals, but either we don't absorb or activate those compounds in the same way when they come in the pill form, or there are other chemical compounds in foods that are the real cancer-fighting ingredients. The list of vitamin supplements that have failed to ward off cancer includes: vitamins B6, B12, E, C, D, beta carotene, folic acid, and selenium.

Pound for Pound, Extra Ones Increase the Risk of Cancer

Excess weight definitely increases the risk of getting cancer, and the reasons are not fully understood. Certainly fat is a very hormonally active substance, and some of those hormones can cause inflammation, which is dry tinder for cancer (human papilloma virus in the cervix is a good example). Fat also increases the levels of estrogen in the body, which might be why it increases the risk of breast cancer in postmenopausal women. Obesity also increases the chance of getting cancer of the esophagus, pancreas, uterus, kidney, thyroid, and gall bladder. That's enough to kill anybody's appetite.

To remember all of these cancer risk factors, picture an obese genital wart, smoking and sipping on a White Russian while lying in a tanning bed in a basement full of radon.

The Revolutions Came with Side Effects

Cancer seems to be everywhere nowadays, so what is going on? Although the Industrial and Chemical Revolutions have generally been very good to us, some of the stuff we cooked up went bad. There are a host of chemicals that we now know are either carcinogenic or unhealthy in other ways; some had industrial applications, some household uses, and some medical (thalidomide, for example). Some we've banned, and some we're still using, with more or less caution.

Our bodies, our cells, our genes are thus being immersed and reimmersed in a changing flux of molecules—pesticides, pharmaceutical drugs, plastics, cosmetics, estrogens, food products, hormones, even novel forms of physical impulses, such as radiation and magnetism. Some of these, inevitably, will be carcinogenic. We cannot wish the world away; our task, then, is to sift through it vigilantly to discriminate bona fide carcinogens from innocent and useful bystanders.

—*Siddhartha Mukherjee,*
The Emperor of All Maladies

They're everywhere. We are surrounded by, and inhale and ingest, the effluent of the Chemical Revolution. That new car smell everyone loves is actually the car exhaling ("off-gassing") volatile organic compounds (VOCs) from the plastics and adhesives used in the car's interior. Those chemicals are not the physiological equivalent of cyanide, a quick death. But there's reason to believe that some of these ubiquitous compounds may increase the risk of bad things happening, including malignant behavior.

Blood testing shows that many of us are carrying around a host of chemical compounds that are not even mentioned in the Original Recipe Book. We don't need them to live, but there they are. In 2016, the Environmental Working Group compiled a comprehensive list of known or likely carcinogens that have been measured in people, and the number came to 420. The idea that man-made chemicals have powerful functions in certain defined applications but suddenly become inert when we ingest or inhale them seems like wishful thinking, or what I call "something-for-nothing science."

The paranoid life is a lonely and fearful one. There's always *something* to worry about. But I prefer a more cautionary, consumer-centered approach to chemicals: prove that it's safe and I'll use it, rather than try it out on the public and pull it from stores shelves later if it ends up being lethal or dangerous.

LUNG CANCER

Like a Bad Houseguest, Too Often Lung Cancer Shows Up Late, Drunk, and Hostile

Behold, the lungs. Every five seconds or so, every day of your life, you take a breath. The diaphragm muscle that separates your chest from your abdomen contracts down, the ribs lift, and air gets sucked in. Traveling through a series of smaller tubes (bronchi, bronchioles), the breath comes to the end of the line in a tiny air sac, an alveolus, where oxygen is offloaded in exchange for carbon dioxide. When the muscles of the diaphragm and ribs relax, we exhale, and then start over. It's a beautiful system, but lung cancer is an ugly disease.

MAN OVERBOARD!

How ugly? As mentioned earlier, lung cancer is roughly half as common as prostate cancer and yet it causes twice as many deaths.

Symptoms of lung cancer

The most common symptoms of lung cancer include cough, chest pain, shortness of breath, weight loss, fatigue, hoarseness, or coughing up blood (or old blood that looks rusty). Sometimes it's a pneumonia or bronchitis that just won't seem to clear. Unfortunately, most lung cancers don't cause any symptoms until the cancer has spread, so there is often no early warning.

Lung cancer is not the most common form of cancer, but it's the leading cause of cancer deaths. Smoking major risk, radon second. All too often, by the time it's found, it's already spread beyond the lung, and then difficult to cure. Surgical removal, chemotherapy, radiation, and newer targeted therapies are treatment options.

Lung Cancer Diagnosis: Getting a Biopsy

As with most cancers, a biopsy will be necessary to confirm the diagnosis. Benign lung tumors do exist (most commonly they are scars from a prior infection) but CT scans are pretty good at deciphering the good from the bad.

There are two ways to get a lung biopsy. A radiologist can use a CT scan to guide a needle between the ribs and into the nodule. Or a pulmonologist, a lung doctor, can do a bronchoscopy, where a flexible fiber-optic tube is guided down the airways of the lung until the tumor is encountered, and then a biopsy is performed through the bronchoscope.

Staging: Tracing the Villain's Footsteps

I like to think of our lungs like a tree: air comes in through a big trunk (the trachea) and then goes through smaller and smaller branches until it reaches the leaves (the air sacs). Lung cancer can start anywhere along the tree. When it spreads, it either grows in place, moves into the lymphatic channels that run along every airway branch and drain back toward the center of the chest, or jumps into the bloodstream to set up camp elsewhere in the body.

There are two main subgroups of lung cancer:

- Small-cell lung cancer makes up 15 percent of all lung cancers, and is almost exclusively caused by smoking.
- Non-small-cell lung cancer (NSCLC) makes up the remaining 85 percent.

Both have a more-than-annoying habit of not alerting us to their presence until they've already spread outside the lungs. By that time, a cure is more difficult, if not impossible. Small-cell cancer is almost always that way (advanced, harder to cure) and NSCLC is a little better. To have a shot of curing NSCLC—which typically involves surgically removing the tumor—we hope to find it before it has moved too deep into the lymphatic system.

That's why looking for possible lymph node involvement is such a critical part of the initial workup. If the biopsy comes back as lung cancer, the next step is to use CT scans, PET imaging, and MRIs to search for clues of wider spread such as enlarged lymph nodes or metastases. Lung cancer has a predilection for going to the brain, bones or liver.

Here's the kicker: although having normal-sized lymph nodes on a CT scan is a good sign, it cannot rule out microscopic disease, and untreated microscopic disease will become macroscopic one day and cause serious issues. Certain regional centers are now combining CT scans and sophisticated computers to create a 3D map of the lung, which is used to steer the bronchoscope to the exact spot needed to biopsy a suspicious tumor. If a quick look at the biopsy suggests lung cancer, biopsies can then be taken of lymph nodes draining that area during the same procedure setting. Since lymph channels run right along the airways, ultrasound can be used to "visualize" the lymph nodes and a needle can be passed through the airway and into the lymph node.

In the old days, the only way to get that kind of information was to have surgery. If you believe *The Crown*'s telling, King George had his left lung removed for lung cancer. Although the king's esteemed surgeon saw that the cancer was already extensively spread, his Royal Highness was not informed of his royally horrible diagnosis until months later, when the truth was becoming patently obvious. Today's complex and technical lymph node biopsies can provide microscopic staging information, critical data that will get surgery to those who can truly benefit, and spare those who would not.

Lung Cancer Treatment

Treating lung cancer can be like the idiom of closing the barn door after the horses have gone. The horses (lung cancer cells) have very often spread out over half the county, well beyond the part of the lung where they were initially stabled. For small-cell lung cancer, the horses have most commonly left the barn: a majority of newly diagnosed patients have metastatic disease– whereas 40 percent of patients with non-small cell lung cancer (NSCLC) show up with metastases.

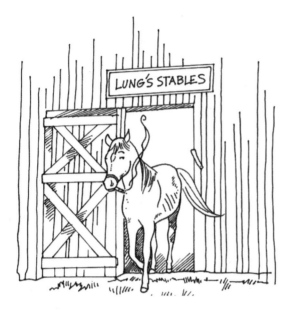

Of course, here's where the simile breaks down, because you're not trying to get these cancerous horses back into the barn. You're trying to kill them, before they kill you.

But NSCLC is not that sensitive to chemotherapy or radiation. Like something out of a Marvel comics movie, these horses are mutant and aggressive, to the point where their normally soft coats are more like Kevlar, and, they *keep…flipping…you…off with one of those one-fingered hoof waves.* It's maddening.

So the best chance of cure comes with surgery, but surgery only makes sense if the tumor isn't too large and it hasn't spread extensively into lymph nodes or critical areas deeper in the chest (termed "regional" disease). On rare occasions, radiation therapy combined with chemotherapy can be curative in someone with early-stage disease who isn't a surgical candidate.

Surgery is what you think it is: a thoracic surgeon removes the portion of the lung with tumors. It's no cakewalk and carries a 3 percent to 5 percent mortality. That's 1 in 20. Testing is done preoperatively to make sure the patient will still be able to breathe adequately after surgery.

For those who are surgical candidates but have more extensive disease, chemotherapy and/or radiation is often used after surgery to lower the serious and substantial risk of recurrence, and to hopefully eliminate whatever microscopic disease the surgeon couldn't get.

Chemo for Lung Cancer: 6 out of 10 on the Shit Sandwich Scale

For those who have extensive lymph node disease or metastases, where cure is not an option, the decision to use chemotherapy balances the time it might buy versus side effects and quality of life. The novel therapies (Opdivo/nivolumab might have the biggest TV footprint) are also being used to try to stop disease progression.

Too often, lung cancer is a horse that cannot be corralled. According to the National Cancer Institute, from 2011 to 2017 the five-year survival rate for those diagnosed with NSCLC was a deeply disappointing 26 percent (64 percent for those with lung-only disease, 37 percent for those with regional spread, and 8 percent for metastatic disease). Ouch. Let's take this moment to give lung cancer the one-hoof wave.

Lung Cancer Screening

It's generally known that either a regular chest X-ray or looking for cancer cells in spit samples is just too crude a tool to use for lung cancer screening.

A CT scan is a much more sophisticated test and can detect a tumor that is just a few millimeters in size. So annual CT scanning using low-dose radiation techniques is now being recommended for those who meet *all three* of these criteria:

- a current smoker or a smoker who quit fewer than 15 years ago
- between the ages of 55 and 80
- who has smoked heavily (more than 30 "pack-years"—multiplying packs per day times years smoked)

The two clinical trials that led to the above recommendations showed a 16 percent and 24 percent reduction in lung cancer deaths. From a lottery standpoint, 303 and 132 people, respectively, needed to be screened to save one life.

Lung Cancer Prevention

Ninety percent of lung cancer in men is caused by smoking. Sadly that includes smoking by proxy, as secondhand smoke increases risk of lung cancer by 20 percent.

The remaining 10 percent is filled out by:
- Radon
- Good old-fashioned air pollution
- Work-related exposure to asbestos, arsenic, beryllium, cadmium, chromium, nickel, and stuffed green peppers (sorry, it's just a personal—not scientific—vendetta)
- Radiation (typically, having had radiation to the chest for breast cancer or lymphoma)

And here's a weird one: high-intensity smokers who take beta-carotene supplements have a higher risk of lung cancer. If you want beta carotene, stick with carrots.

19 COLORECTAL CANCER

The Lowly GI System, and the Little Polyp That Could—but Hopefully Won't

As organ systems go, the gastrointestinal (GI) system has always been treated like a double-A farm team, a journeyman organ whose career path does not end at the big leagues with the heart or the brain. We think of it as a rather mindless conveyor belt coursing down the middle of us, where anything of food value is pulled off the conveyor belt, and what's left over is waste.

Proof of its ignominious stature is the fact that many GI terms have a tone of immodest indecency that make Cub Scouts smile and mothers scowl. Anus. Rectum. Sphincter. Hemorrhoid. Feces. Poop. Shit. See? These terms have a cultural, emotional value that you don't find in terms like right atrium, meniscus, ureter, or temporal lobe.

But research is showing us that the GI system is incredibly complex and highly sophisticated, a nod to the undeniable fact that if you can't absorb what you eat, you're dead. So hats off, please, and hands over your abdomen (not your heart) as we pause for a moment of respect for this unsung hero of undeserved ignominy, this organ system with the longstanding shitty reputation.

MAN OVERBOARD!

If found early, as a cancerous polyp on the inside of colon, colorectal cancer can be cured by snipping it out during colonoscopy. The deeper it grows into the wall of the colon—or beyond—the harder it is to cure. Even so, it's considerably "friendlier" than lung cancer. Surgery, chemotherapy are treatment mainstays.

Time's up. Unfortunately, we're not here to sing its praises, but rather to probe the GI system's dark side. Cancer can and does arise anywhere in the GI tract, but most commonly it develops at the end of the line: the colon ("large intestine") and the rectum. The large intestine meets the small intestine at the level of our beltline on the right side of the abdomen, then courses up toward the chest, across the lower edge of the ribs, then down the left side of the abdomen and finally into the pelvis.

Poop-Chute Cancer: Where Does It Start, How Does It Grow?

Although there are many different types of cells in the GI system—glandular, smooth muscle, nerves, hormonal—most colorectal cancers begin in the cells that make up the inner lining. They begin as a benign overgrowth of tissue—a polyp—that starts out rather flat and then forms a knuckle or finger of tissue.

It takes a polyp 10 years or more to go from benign to cancerous, and usually the cancerous cells are found at the tip of the polyp. At this early stage, a polyp with cancer can often be completely removed during a colonoscopy, and the patient can be cured.

Left to its own malignant devices, the cancer will go on a bender and stumble down into the stalk of the polyp, then into the base of the polyp, and then into the colon itself. How far it gets before being discovered is the basis for the staging system used in colorectal cancer.

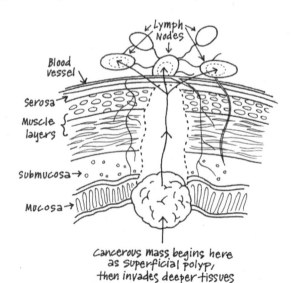

Cancerous mass begins here as superficial polyp, then invades deeper tissues

MAN OVERBOARD!

- Stage 0: The cancer just involves the inside lining of the colon.
- Stage 1: It's moved into the colon wall.
- Stage 2: The cancer now involves the full thickness of the colon wall, and may have moved into the fat surrounding the colon.
- Stage 3: The cancer has gotten into lymph nodes.
- Stage 4: It's spread into another organ ("metastasized," a word that puts a lump in the throat of every doctor who has to utter it). Most commonly the other organ is the liver, because almost all of the blood from the GI tract drains to the liver first before heading back to the heart for recirculation.

Colon cancer is often a symptomless disease. It's not until the cancer is very advanced and bulky that it can plug things up and cause abdominal pain, bloating, or obvious blood in the stool. In fact, sometimes it's not discovered until it has spread and begins causing painful stretching of the liver.

Treatment for Fartbag Cancer

You can see this coming: the farther and deeper the cancer goes, the more trouble it is.

A small cancerous polyp can be removed easily and completely by a Jedi warrior armed with a light saber, or more typically by a GI doctor armed with a colonoscope that can either snip or snare the polyp. If the polyp is small and the cancer superficial, its removal usually portends a complete cure. But if the cancer has been around long enough to grow into the colon wall or beyond, you'll need surgery. That means cutting out the part of the colon containing the cancer, along with some lymph nodes. As with many types of cancer-removal surgery, tissue samples from the operating room are quickly frozen and analyzed by a pathologist so that the surgeon can know how much colon and how many lymph nodes to remove. Then, just like you did after you ran over the extension cord with a lawnmower, the surgeon reconnects the two loose ends of the colon so that the patient once again has a contiguous, glorious tubular conveyor belt for food.

Following surgery, patients with cancer in the lymph nodes or other high risk features will be treated with chemotherapy (or sometimes radiation) to try to eliminate any rogue cells that were hiding out and evaded the scalpel.

Chemo for Colon Cancer: 5 out of 10 on the Shit Sandwich Scale

If you needed proof that colorectal cancer is less aggressive than lung cancer, here it is: *some* patients with metastatic disease, limited to the liver or lung, have a 25 percent chance of being cured with surgery. By "some" I mean there can't be too many tumors, and they have to be in a place where they can be safely removed, and the patient has to have enough liver or lung to live on after the procedure. It's not an easy club to join because there are a paltry number of cancers in which the words "metastatic" and "cure" can peacefully coexist in the same sentence.

As with many other cancers, there is an ever-expanding number of novel therapies that can block critical metabolic or immune pathways in colon cancer. There are no home runs yet—a single, maybe a stretch double—and they are only being used in patients with advanced disease. Remember, Rome wasn't built in a day—but then the Romans didn't have the kind of research dollars that Big Pharma has.

A Word on Rectal Cancer

The rectum is the last stop on the stool train, if you don't count the anus. When the rectum gets distended with stool, it sends a message to the upstream colon to begin a series of organized contractions that doctors call "peristalsis" and regular people call "the urge." It also sends a message to the two sphincters (muscular valves, really) in the anal canal. They'll need to relax and open when the timing is right.

Here's one thing that rectal cancer has in common with real estate: location, location, location. Although rectal cancer develops like colon cancer, the rectum is buried deep in the pelvis, with the sacrum (the shovel-shaped end of the spine where the butt cheeks attach) on one side and the bladder and prostate gland on the other.

It's in a tight location, making it difficult to remove surgically. If you've ever done an engine repair where the job itself is straightforward, but the access is nearly impossible, you'll know what a surgeon is up against. So any rectal cancer that involves the bowel wall or lymph nodes requires a combination of radiation, chemotherapy, and surgery. And it's possible that the patient will end up with a permanent colostomy, where the colon is sewed to the abdominal wall, and stool collects in a bag.

Is This Serious Doo-Doo?

How serious is colorectal cancer? Plenty serious, but better than lung cancer. The five-year survival rate is 90 percent for those with localized disease, 73 percent for those with lymph node or regional spread, and 15 percent for those with metastatic disease. Cancer is a trickster and a villain, so the word "cure" is used cautiously, but the National Cancer Institute claims that 50 percent of those with localized disease can be cured with surgery.

Colon Cancer Screening

As mentioned previously, polyps that develop in the lining of the colon take 8 to 10 years to turn cancerous.

The idea of screening for colon cancer is to find polyps early in that decade-long process. When to start screening depends on your risk, but people of average risk should probably get started at age 45. Here's the list of screening options.

Microscopic Blood in the Stool

The simplest screening test is to check several stool samples for microscopic amounts of blood. There are two varieties: guaiac fecal occult blood test (FOBT) or fecal immunochemical test (FIT). (Oddly enough, obvious amounts of blood in the stool are rarely due to cancer, but are more likely due to hemorrhoids or something called "diverticulosis.") The sampling process required by these tests give you the chance to interact with your stool in an entirely new way, which in itself is an enriching life experience.

Microscopic Blood and Cancer Gene Fragments in the Stool

The Cologuard (FIT-DNA) is a stool test that combines the FIT test described above and a test that detects colorectal cancer-associated DNA fragments. The combination makes it better at finding cancer or larger polyps than a FIT or FOBT test alone, but it carries a higher chance of giving a false positive result, which might well lead to a colonoscopy.

Flexible Sigmoidoscopy

Statistically speaking, most colon cancers develop in the sigmoid colon, the last part of the colon, which can be directly visualized by inserting a flexible sigmoidoscope up the hinder. A "flex sig" is a fiber-optic scope that can be nimbly steered by the operator as it is threaded up the sigmoid. Some people's sigmoid colons can have more twists and turns than a high mountain road, and for those patients, the flex sig may not feel so flexible. The procedure takes about 15 minutes and doesn't typically require sedation.

Colonoscopy

Colonoscopy is the same sort of technology as a flex sig, but the scope is longer—about 5 feet. So when it's brought into the room by technicians, it may look to you like one of those dragons in a Chinese New Year parade.

A colonoscopy can visualize the entire colon, but it's a more complicated and lengthy procedure than a flex sig, and it requires some level of sedation. While colonoscopy clearly does detect more polyps, simply because it looks at more of the colon, at this point there is only indirect evidence that colonoscopy lowers colon cancer mortality when compared with flex-sig screening (trials are underway). It does, however, unequivocally raise the cost of health care.

CT Colonography ("Virtual Colonoscopy")

You'll hear news reports about "virtual colonoscopy," which is a colonoscopy done via a CT scanner. It sounds like welcome news to those people with zigzagging sigmoid colons that make a regular colonoscopy challenging, but the technology isn't quite there yet, and even if it does find a polyp, then what? That's right. You'll need a traditional colonoscopy to have it removed.

Just Pick One

A CDC report noted that in 2018 about 30 percent of eligible adults were not up to date with their colon cancer screening, and those in their early 50s were the most likely to be unscreened. That information, coupled with a 15 percent increase in colorectal cancer in people in their 40's since the year 2000, led the US Preventive Services Task Force (USPSTF) to lower the age criteria for screening. They concluded that screening adults aged 45-49 offered moderate certainty of moderate benefits, and that continuing to screen those aged 50 to 75 years offered a high certainty of substantial benefit.

When it comes to screening for colorectal cancer, the USPSTF has a very pragmatic recommendation: those who have never been screened are the most likely to benefit, so just pick one. Please. Just get started.

Colorectal Cancer Prevention

The best thing you can do to avoid colon cancer is to avoid excessive use of alcohol and don't smoke. Avoid excess weight, moderate the amount of red meat you eat, and load up on fruits and vegetables, particularly cruciferous vegetables. The list includes broccoli, Brussels sprouts, arugula, and cauliflower, among others; these plants are the rock stars of the nutrition world, without any of the chemical dependency issues. Cruciferous vegetables are high in glucosinolates, a type of chemical that might be part of the cancer-lowering effect of these famously fibrous foods.

If you're not open to arugula and bok choy, how about a baby aspirin every other day? No one knows exactly how an aspirin might work to prevent cancer, but aspirin does prevent inflammation, and chronic inflammation seems to be fertile ground for the development of cancer.

Two large studies showing that long term, regular aspirin use reduced colorectal cancer by 19% led to a recommendation in 2016 by the US Preventive Services Task Force (USPSTF) for low-dose aspirin use in people in their 50's who were not at increased risk of bleeding, and who were willing to stick with it for 10 years. But by 2022, additional, less favorable trial results caused the USPSTF to pull that recommendation. So for now, skip the aspirin and continue grazing on rutabaga and Chinese cabbage and also the neighbor's lawn clippings, as long as they're cruciferous.

20 PROSTATE CANCER

The King of Male Cancers; Wanna Buy a PSA Powerball Ticket?

The "his" and "hers" of cancer are undoubtedly prostate and breast cancer, and their unfortunate commonness has made them a regular part of our lives, with marquee events like Movember and multiday breast cancer walks.

Breasts serve an obvious biological role—feeding infants—and they occupy a high-profile position on the female body, both anatomically and sexually. The prostate gland's location deep within the pelvis makes it a much more reclusive organ than the female breast. That's probably why it hasn't spawned a multibillion-dollar fashion industry, with a flagship company called Bernie's Secret, and why women aren't free to comment on the shape, size, geographical positioning, and symmetry of men's prostate glands.

Oddly enough, both organs are associated with uncomfortable, contortionist screening tests: the breast gets flattened to quesadilla thickness for a mammogram, and men get a finger up the rectum for a prostate check (an exam maneuver perhaps most fa-

MAN OVERBOARD!

The majority of men, if they live long enough, will develop prostate cancer, but what kind will it be? The most common kind—a sleepy, slow-growing version that dawdles along well into geezerhood? Or the aggressive kind that can strike and kill pre-geezers? Biopsies and PSAs have been a murky crystal ball.

To treat or not to treat, that is the question: one's age and underlying health conditions are important considerations. Treatment involves surgical removal or radiation, with similar outcomes but different potential complications. If cancer is widespread, starve it of testosterone to hold it in check.

mously canonized by Chevy Chase in the movie *Fletch*. Singing a line from "Moon River," Fletch then says, "Thank you Doc. Ever serve time?"; "Using the whole fist, Doc?"). This so-called "digital exam" (the digit being a finger, not a numeric symbol) works because the prostate gland sits right in front of the rectum, below the bladder, and surrounds the urethra as it exits the bladder and funnels out into the penis.

Like your average dog, the prostate gland spends enormous amounts of time just lounging around, with fitful and brief periods of intense action. For the prostate, the action part comes during orgasm. It's the job of the prostate to secrete a thin milky fluid that serves as an "adventure pack" for the sperm as they come flying by on their way out to the Promised Land. The "adventure pack" includes some glue so that the semen can stick to the cervix, but also a slow-release glue dissolver, which allows the sperm to eventually swim free of the cervix and begin the ultimate swimming competition up into the uterus.

The prostate of a young male is the size of a walnut in the shell, but as men age, it's common for it to slowly grow, sometimes to the size of a lemon. We call that "hypertrophy" in medicalese, as in benign prostatic hypertrophy (BPH). As the prostate increases in size, it often crimps the urethra, which crimps urination and also the ability of the bladder to completely empty itself, which then crimps sleep as the owner drags himself off to the bathroom several times a night. What an odd thing, that a generous prostate gland can put bags under your eyes.

Having BPH doesn't increases one's chances of prostate cancer or having sexual problems, but it can sure complicate life. Treatment options include these two medications: alpha blockers, which relax the muscles in the bladder and prostate and thereby improve urine flow; and drugs like finasteride, which we discussed in the hair loss chapter. Finasteride blocks the conversion of testosterone to DHT: this allows hair follicles to grow, and causes prostate glands to shrink.

What about Saul Palmetto, the guy who played second base for the '49 Yankees? Or rather saw palmetto, a shrub-sized palm whose fruit is used to create a supplement that's been widely used for BPH? If it works for you, then let your experience inform you, because the science can't back you up. Two large high-quality studies funded by the National Institutes of Health showed saw palmetto to be a swing and a miss.

If medications don't work, several types of surgical therapies can remove excess prostate tissue and open things up.

Prostate Cancer: Not So Much "If," but More Like "When and What Kind?"

As if whizzing issues and sleep deprivation weren't enough, the prostate sometimes tries to kill us. With the Big C, cancer. The problem with prostate cancer is that it often doesn't fit our definition of cancer. For most men, it will be a slow-growing, couch potato kind of cancer, an almost "benign" kind of cancer (as odd as that sounds).

Proof of its typically slothful character is the fact that autopsy studies show a steady age-related increase in the percentage of men with cancerous changes in their prostate glands. One study found microscopic amounts of prostate cancer in 27 percent of men in the 30 to 39 age range, and in 34 percent of men ages 40 to 49. Another autopsy study on men who died after age 60, of something other than prostate cancer, found that more than half of them had prostate cancer, and the likelihood only rises with age.

The question then really isn't "Who will get prostate cancer?" because the majority of men will if they live long enough. The question is what *kind* of prostate cancer will he get: the untroubling, sleepy "benign" form, or the uncommon but more aggressive and deadly form? And if it is the "benign" form, could he live long enough that it might one day grow to the size where it would give him trouble? This is what makes prostate cancer screening so complicated and controversial.

Prostate Cancer Growth, Diagnosis, Staging

Prostate cancer typically begins in the periphery of the prostate gland, not in the prostate's core, where the urethra goes through. That explains why a tinkling urinary stream, slow bladder emptying, dribbling at the end of urination, or waking up at night to pee are symptoms more likely caused by *benign* prostatic hypertrophy (BPH) than cancer (and by the simple statistical fact that BPH is far more common than cancer). It's also why a prostate exam can detect cancerous bumps (nodules) on the outside of the prostate and it's the explanation for why men can sometimes have few to no prostate cancer symptoms until it has spread into the bones.

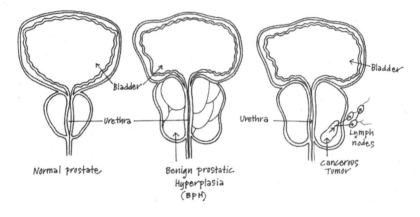

Like lung and colon cancers, prostate cancer begins locally and then slowly makes its way through the prostate's outer lining (the capsule), then to lymph nodes, and then rides the bloodstream to metastasize into the bones.

If a rising blood level of prostate-specific antigen (PSA, detailed later in this chapter) or the presence of a prostate nodule raises the question of cancer, the answer will likely come in the form a transrectal ultrasound-guided biopsy (TRUS). As the name squeamishly suggests, a urologist—a surgeon specializing in the kidneys, bladder, and prostate—will convert your rectum into a shooting gallery, generally under sedation. Using ultrasound as a visual guide, the urologist uses a hollow needle to remove a core of tissue from the prostate. He or she may home in on a suspicious-looking area, or take scattered samples (generally 10-12 in total). Then you're free to wander the midway with the impossibly large and ugly stuffed animal that you won.

Alternatively, an MRI machine can provide the clearest and most detailed images of the prostate and surrounding tissues, and like ultrasound, it can be used to guide biopsies. In what sounds like a science experiment gone horribly wrong, sometimes a probe that emits radio waves is inserted up the hinder to further enhance the images.

If you're lucky and the pathologist finds no cancer in the biopsies, the question remains whether the biopsies were taken from the right places; and for that reason, at some point in the future the urologist or radiologist will want to go traipsing back up your rectum.

. If you're unlucky and the pathologist finds cancer in the biopsies, they will rate how malignant (how irregular, twisted, or abnormal) the cells look and then give it a Gleason score. Like golf, a good score is low, and a high score is bad. A Gleason score of 6 or lower (out of 10) is considered a low grade.

If you've been paying attention—and why wouldn't you be?— you're probably thinking that the next step is to try to see if the cancer has spread out of the prostate and into local lymph nodes, or into any other areas. And you would be correct.

You're probably also thinking that the Gleason score, and the PSA level, and the results of the radiology tests would be used to put people into different prostate cancer stages, so we could match best treatment options for that stage. Correct again.

Stage 1:   cancer only in prostate, with low Gleason and PSA
Stage 2:   cancer still confined to prostate, but involving more of it, with increasing Gleason and PSA
Stage 3:   some combination of worrisome factors, like very high PSA, or growth into local tissues (rectum, bladder, pelvic wall)
Stage 4a: shoot, it's into the pelvic lymph nodes
Stage 4b: spread to bones or distant lymph nodes

Prostate Cancer Treatment

If you end up getting diagnosed with prostate cancer, *do not panic*. In most cases, prostate cancer is the not-so-cancerous cancer. As a 2020 article in the *New England Journal of Medicine* put it, "Most PSA-detected prostate cancers thus act more like a chronic disease than an aggressive malignancy." The five-year relative survival rate for those diagnosed with localized prostate cancer is 100 percent. And even more remarkably, it's 100 percent for those whose cancer had spread into lymph nodes. Now, survival rates are not cure rates, and it's possible that the typically slow-growing prostate cancer could show up sometime later. But hopefully much, much later.

Before reviewing treatment options, there are a couple of key questions to ask.

What Kind of Prostate Cancer Do I Have, and How Should I Feel about It?

Most PSA-detected prostate cancers are low grade and localized to the prostate, in which case, there's no emergency. You have time to think this through. It might be entirely reasonable just to watch what's happening with your PSA over time, hum an occasional "Moon River," repeat a biopsy in a year, and if it hasn't changed, space out the biopsies further. This approach is often called "watchful waiting."

Although a diagnosis of low-grade prostate cancer may be the best version of some bad news, it's hardly a relief. The doctor can't say with absolute certainty that the cancer won't flip a genetic switch and turn ugly, and besides, it's not our instinct to want to *live with* cancer. It's a burden. We've been well taught to go to war with cancer. We want it out. Take it out with surgery. Nuke it with radiation. We all want to be cancer free.

When faced with a "Gandhi vs. Ultimate Fighter" kind of cancer choice, men often choose the more aggressive option. They're not interested in nonviolent protest, so-called "watchful waiting." They want to beat the crap out of it with a series of leg whips. In this way, a trip down the PSA trail commonly leads to prostate cancer treatment.

How Much Calendar Time Do You Think You Have Left?

As we grow older, finance experts recommend that we pull our savings out of the stock market and put it into bonds. The investment window is short: you have less time to rebound from a correction. Similarly, older men with prostate cancer have less to gain and more to lose by pursuing aggressive prostate therapies.

I once took care of a man who, at 86 years old, got radiation therapy for his newly discovered prostate cancer (personally and professionally, I would not recommend looking for trouble—or an elevated PSA—at that age). He wound up being unlucky enough to get radiation damage to his bladder, and spent his remaining years in a fog of sleep deprivation from having to drain his bladder every two hours. Not good.

In my experience, people often presume that they will almost certainly reach the age of their parents, or beyond that given the wonders of modern medicine. Don't bet on it. Our parents, and particularly our grandparents, grew up in much different environments, and were often much heartier. They didn't grow up with excess calories, they weren't exposed to the environmental toxins we have been ("Oh, that used car smell!"), couldn't afford cigarettes, and they really did walk two miles uphill—both ways—to school. The wonders of modern medicine are in direct competition with the unhealthy aspects of modern life. Some days it's not clear which one is winning.

In any case, "How much time do I have left?" is a hard question to ask and a hard one to answer, even for a physician. But if you've been diagnosed with prostate cancer, coming up with a ballpark estimate will help you make some decisions.

How Healthy Are You?

Of course, how healthy you are has a lot of say about how long you might live.

I grew up on the edge of farm country in northern Illinois. I went to tractor pull competitions, where a tractor pulls a sled down a straightaway against an ever-increasing amount of weight (when I was a kid this was men spaced at regular intervals on both sides of the track, and they'd jump on as the sled passed. Now the sled has a cantilevered weight that automatically gets "heavier"). The idea was for the tractor to get as far down the track as possible before it literally stopped in its tracks.

Life is a tractor pull. The load gets heavier as one goes. You go until the tires slip or the transmission blows near the grandstand. If you have a lot of baseline medical problems weighing you down, aggressive care might offer you all of the risks and none of the benefits.

If you've discussed the questions with your physician and feel like pursuing treatment, here are the three main treatment options.

Surgery: Get Rad' with a Radical Prostatectomy

A radical prostatectomy involves removing the prostate gland, the seminal vesicles, and probably lymph nodes. As I mentioned, the pelvis is a complicated place to perform surgery: zero headroom and a lot of important things—rectum, bladder, major arteries, and nerves heading off to the legs—stuffed into the bony cage of the pelvis.

The main risks of a prostatectomy are the droops (erectile dysfunction, ED) and the dribbles (urinary incontinence). This is thought to be primarily from injury to the hoisting nerve and the wiz valve nerve. Certain surgical approaches are touted as "nerve sparing," but results may have more to do with the skill and patience of the surgeon than the approach.

Both the droops and the dribbles are very common *immediately* after surgery, but most men show significant improvement over time. Even so, two years after surgery 40 percent of men have erectile dysfunction, and 5 percent to 10 percent have chronic, moderate-to-severe incontinence.

Radiation

Radiation treatment keeps a surgeon from mucking around in one's pelvis, and avoids some of the attendant risks of anesthesia and post-op complications. For men with other significant medical issues, this might make radiation the obvious choice. But radiation faces some of the same challenges as surgery in terms of working in a crowded pelvis. The goal is to "nuke" the prostate without injuring the neighbors—primarily the bladder and the rectum. If those get burned, the inner lining of either can break down and bleed, and injury to the muscles and nerves can cause spasms of the bladder or rectum that are both painful and sometimes entirely too spontaneous, if you know what I mean. Fortunately these are generally short-term side effects, and affect only a very small percentage of men chronically. Radiation also carries the risk of dribbling, and the risk of erectile dysfunction is perhaps as high as 60 percent to 70 percent—but that may be because the medical issues that pushed men to choose radiation over surgery also put them at higher risk of ED.

Radiation can be delivered externally, in what's called a "beam," or delivered internally, by planting radioactive seeds into the prostate.

Hormone Therapy

The main treatment option for metastatic prostate cancer is depriving the tumor of androgens (the male hormones, like testosterone—hence the term "androgen deprivation therapy"). Castration does that quickly and cheaply and is a common approach in many parts of the world. If you want to keep your balls, we can use medications to shut the gonads off ("chemical castration"), keeping them for decorative effect even while starving the cancer of androgens.

Of course, that means the rest of the body is without androgens too, so male menopause symptoms follow: loss of muscle, fatigue, erectile dysfunction, decreased libido, hot flashes, a little breast development. Long-term risks include blood clots in the veins and osteoporosis, and possible increased risk of cardiovascular disease.

Although almost all prostate cancers respond well to androgen deprivation therapy, eventually—usually years later—the cancer cells figure out a way around it. Cancer cells divide at a fast rate, and the process is bungling and littered with genetic errors. But sometimes one of those "errors" is the winning lottery ticket for the cancer—that is, a new line of prostate cancer cells that don't require androgen stimulation to grow. That happens with chemotherapy, too: a cancer that was previously held in check by treatment X may begin to grow again.

Prostate Cancer Screening and the PSA

The oldest prostate cancer screening test—a finger up the hinder—allowed the doctor to feel the outside of the prostate gland for any irregularities or bumps. (Doctors use the term "prostate nodules" because it sounds more technical and better justifies the discomfort of the exam.)

Unfortunately, this prostate exam via the rectum hasn't proven to be a particularly refined way of finding cancer. It is very operator dependent, and as one might think, it only detects more advanced, macroscopic cancers, not early, microscopic disease. Like the breast self-exam, opinions are often stronger than science as to whether it's worth doing.

And then, in 1994, the FDA approved the PSA (prostate-specific antigen) test for use in screening asymptomatic men for prostate cancer. PSA is a protein secreted at low levels by normal prostate cells, and more vigorously by malignant cells. PSA levels tend to rise with age as the prostate increases in size, during infections of the prostate (prostatitis), and with prostate cancer. PSAs tend to run lower in those with increased body fat (raising questions about whether the normal range should vary based on obesity), and they generally fall by 50% for patients taking finasteride or dutasteride for benign prostatic hypertrophy. That makes sense, since a shrinking prostate will make less PSA. Taking these drugs can make using PSA levels for prostate cancer a little tricky. As a rule of thumb, it's recommended that anyone taking finasteride or dutasteride should double his PSA value before comparing it to normal (4 ng/dl), and any sharp uptick in PSA should be watched closely.

In an effort to squeeze more clinical meaning out of the PSA test, various PSA spin-offs have been created such as the "free PSA," the "PSA velocity" (how fast is it rising over time), the "Pro-PSA," and my personal favorites: the "Bernie's Secret PSA," the "Black and Decker 5-in-1 PSA," and the "Talladega Super Speedway Sprint Cup Series PSA." None of these has added a lot of clarity to the picture, although the "Black and Decker 5-in-1 PSA" is amazingly versatile and can be used as a miniature jaws-of-life device or as a handy nail file.

Elevated PSA? Three Basic Options

Ignore It

This is *an option*, but, but if it's your preference (and it's an entirely reasonable one for certain people), a better approach might be to not test at all. If ignorance is bliss, embrace it. Don't go halfway.

Recheck It

There is some physiologic "slop" in a PSA value—it can bounce around a little—so typically it would just be rechecked in a couple months, unless the level really jumped up or there are other alarming symptoms.

Get Imaging and a Biopsy

If you want to know more, the next step is an ultrasound or MRI-guided needle biopsy.

The PSA Powerball Lottery
What Do You Need to Wager to Enter, and What Are the Odds of Winning?

You can think of getting your PSA checked more or less like entering a lottery. You pay your money and hope that you'll be one of the winners.

The winning part is obvious: you hope that the screening process will save you from dying of prostate cancer. That would be an easy decision if prostate cancer was uniformly lethal—like a bullet through the heart—and screening was like a bulletproof vest. But that is rarely the case, and a bulletproof vest is a lot to commit to if there are no bullets flying.

The money part is less obvious: in this lottery, you are not handing over $10 to a convenience store clerk. You are handing over your body. You are saying "yes" to the possible complications of what PSA screening could bring to you:

- The discomfort and possible complications of prostate biopsies
- The risks of surgery itself, and post-op problems of droops and dribbles
- The side effects of radiation and the risks of collateral damage to the bladder or the colon
- The mental struggles of being diagnosed with cancer, even a common and less-threatening form like prostate cancer

All of those go into the kitty, and you must be prepared to deal with them to have a chance of winning.

What Are the Odds of Winning the PSA Powerball Lottery?

Three large studies—the PLCO trial in America, the CAP trial in the United Kingdom, and the ERSPC trial in Europe—have given us some real-life insights (as real as any clinical trial can be) into this PSA Powerball.

In 2018, the US Preventive Services Task Force (USPSTF) reviewed the most recent updates from the three trials. The ERSPC trial had the most favorable results: at 13 years of follow-up there was a 30 percent reduction in the number of men who developed metastatic prostate cancer, and a 20 percent drop in prostate cancer mortality. Unfortunately, there was no change in overall mortality: the number of men who ducked prostate cancer was offset by those who died of something else instead. The PLSO (14 years of follow-up) and the CAP trial (10 years of follow-up) didn't demonstrate any prostate cancer mortality benefit.

A prostate cancer mortality reduction of 20 percent is welcome news, and it sounds like a big deal, but as you've heard me caution before, a large percentage of a small number is still a small number. So to help men personalize the trial data, the USPSTF used the benefits observed in these three large trials and sketched out what kind of a gamble one might be taking when buying a PSA Powerball ticket.

If We Screened *1,000 Men* Ages 55 to 69 Every Couple Years with a PSA, and Followed Them for 13 Years

- 240 would have a positive PSA test result
- 220 would end up getting one or more prostate biopsies
- 100 men would be diagnosed with prostate cancer
- 80 men would choose to be treated with surgery or radiation. Of those, 50 would develop erectile dysfunction and 15 would have urinary incontinence.

If that's what a ticket "costs," what's to be won?

- One to two (1.3 to be exact) men would avoid dying of prostate cancer
- Three men would avoid having their prostate cancer metastasize into their bones

MAN OVERBOARD!

A wasted ticket?

- 5 men would die of prostate cancer anyway
- 200 men would die of something other than prostate cancer

Since then, the ERSPC published more encouraging follow-up data, showing that screening 570 men over 16 years would save one life. Could you run a successful Kickstarter-in-the-Pelvis campaign to recruit 570 men to agree to PSA screening in order for one of them to be spared from dying of prostate cancer over a 16-year period?

A 2020 piece in the *New England Journal of Medicine* concurred with the USPSTF recommendation against PSA screening but acknowledged that it's really a value proposition—what do you get for your "money"?—and there's no single right answer.

If it is of any help, I can tell you that male doctors struggle with this on a personal level, the science be damned.

When to Saddle Up for a Ride Down the PSA Trail

There are a number of groups besides the US Preventive Services Task Force that make recommendations on prostate cancer screening, including the American Cancer Society, the American College of Physicians, and the American Urological Association.

Their guidelines vary a bit, but generally they recommend that men ages 50 to 69 have a discussion with their doctor about what to do. Perhaps sooner if you have a father or brother with prostate cancer.

One of the things that committees and task forces do is generate complex-sounding phrases to describe simple things. Here, the term for hashing this PSA stuff out with your doctor has been termed "shared decision making." The opposite of this is "unshared decision making," wherein your doctor straps you to the exam table and draws your PSA.

Deal Me In

I am a child of this PSA quagmire. My father went down the PSA road at age 59, had low-grade cancer on biopsies, and had his prostate surgically removed. His PSA never *quite* went down to zero like it should have, either because they left a little of the prostate gland behind or because the cancer had already spread outside the prostate. For 18 years after the surgery, he watched his PSA slowly rise, and the likelihood of his dying of prostate cancer loomed over everything. It occupied his mind. He understood that prostate cancer commonly spreads to bones, and so every ache and pain had the potential to be the first sign of a cancer that was still hanging around.

And then he developed a fast-moving case of lung cancer and died. The autopsy he requested showed no sign of prostate cancer, but it must have been there on some microscopic level.

So I have a family history of prostate cancer. I'm at increased risk for the disease, but if I get it, is there any guarantee that it would be the kind my father had—a tumor that left the prostate quickly but grew extremely slowly?

Prostate Cancer Prevention

The two main risk factors for prostate cancer—being male and getting older—don't lend themselves to any *reasonable* action plan. Having a father, brother, or son with prostate cancer increases the risk of getting diagnosed with prostate cancer from 8 percent in the general US population to 15 percent, but it's not clear what that means. It may be that those with a family history of prostate cancer end up looking for it more aggressively, and the more you look, the more you find. The risk of dying from prostate cancer is highest among Black men, but this probably has more to do with access to health care than any genetic predisposition.

Japanese natives seem to have the lowest incidence of prostate cancer, but it's likely that the reasons are cultural rather than genetic, because within two generations, Japanese Americans have the same risk as the rest of the population. The difference might be related to dietary fat intake, although this is a highly debated, contentious area, with studies being split, and authoritative entities like the National Cancer Institute describing the relationship between fat intake and prostate cancer as "complex." *If* there is any cause and effect, it must be small, and it is more likely related to saturated fats. In keeping with that, there is some association between higher intake of dairy foods and calcium and prostate cancer, but if it's real, it is small.

A couple of weirdo outtakes: vitamin E supplementation seemed to increase the risk of prostate cancer, as did folate supplementation. But elevated folate levels from dietary intake of folic acid seemed to be protective. Go figure.

You'll notice there are a lot of "mights" and "maybes" in this section on avoiding prostate cancer. You *might* consider not getting older, and if you're going to have a lot of dairy foods like ice cream, you *might* do better choosing something like Ben & Jerry's "Chunky Liver Bits with Spinach Swirls," two foods which have a lot of natural folate in them.

21 MIND GAMES

Mental Health Finally Gets Its Due. Turns Out, Everyone Struggles: Some More, Some Less

I was born in 1965 in the Land of Lincoln. My parents didn't have a parenting philosophy outside of "Go to school. Be home by dinner. Make something of yourself. Leave your brother alone." Although I felt deeply loved and cared for, it was a "PB & J with apple and chips" physical world. What you saw was all there was.

School was readin', writin', and 'rithmetic. The teachers weren't there to raise our emotional IQ. Church was mostly about benevolence (the poor, the sick, the hungry) and redemption (how to avoid becoming extra crispy in the lake of fire). Only salvation could bring inner peace. Doubts, fears, worries, struggles were courtesy of the Other Guy, not God, and should be opposed by prayer.

When it came to male role models, it appeared that action heroes and professional athletes were what I should be shooting for. Contemplative, introspective men like Gandhi, Henry David Thoreau, or Mr. Rogers were no match for steely men of action like John Wayne, James Bond, or Starsky & Hutch. The budding writer

MAN OVERBOARD!

Mood issues such as anxiety and depression are the most common mental health problems by far. You can struggle with symptoms of anxiety or depression without having a full-fledged "disorder." Therapists help untangle dysfunctional thought loops. Medications put brain neurochemistry back in balance. Drug and alcohol abuse are often complicating factors. Yes, mental health issues can profoundly affect quality of life, but risk of suicide means it can sometimes be a lethal illness.

John-Boy on the TV series *The Waltons* was the only male who seemed willing to wrestle with his innermost thoughts and feelings. Strange things happen in the hills of Appalachia.

I was not emotionally suppressed as a boy, but if there were such things as emotions, it seemed as if girls got most of them. Like braids, long hair, jump rope—that was their thing.

My father's father died in an accident when my dad was eight. I asked him a number of times how the tragic loss affected him, and the answer—"I don't know, I was just a kid"—always ended the conversation. His answer may have been a lie or a dodge, but I suspect it was simply the message he was given: "suck it up," "stay strong"—the usual bullshit young men were often reared on.

The Mentally Ill Are Insane and Everyone Else Is Normal

Within this emotional and "inner life" vacuum, the only people I knew who were experiencing mental illness were cooped up in a state mental hospital a couple of towns upriver from my hometown. We rarely drove past its sprawling thousand-plus-acre campus, but when we did, it was spooky, a collection of ancient brick buildings that made it look like Dracula University. (What did commencement look like—capes over capes?) The message was clear: mental health applied to the insane and occurred at a distance, to someone else.

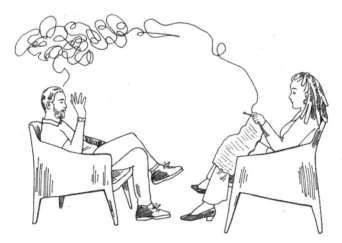

If you didn't grow up near a state mental hospital, and I'm guessing you didn't, then your only other exposure to mental health issues was probably through the TV or movies, where deranged criminality sells. If serial killers such as the paranoid schizophrenic Son of Sam or Jeffrey Dahmer with his borderline personality disorder were in short supply, we could count on Hollywood to fill the gap with characters like Hannibal Lecter, whose struggles with homicidal cannibalism were hardly meant to be a public service announcement for antisocial personality disorder. We were to be titillated and entertained.

All of this had the effect of making relatively uncommon mental health diagnoses seem more like the norm, and also far more criminal than they are. When in actuality, the most common mental health issues are mood disorders like anxiety and depression. The vast majority of those struggling with their mental health are not insisting that T-Mobile, or the Pope, or their long-since-dead high school English teacher is controlling the voices in their heads. They are wondering if they will ever feel like smiling again, or if the (apparent) calmness they see in others will ever be theirs.

Everyone Struggles with Their Mental Health—Some More, Some Less

According to the National Alliance on Mental Illness, 16 million American adults live with serious depression, and 42 million live with an anxiety disorder. That makes anxiety and depression far and away the leading mental health issues, and it's not uncommon to have some mix of the two. It's depressing to always feel anxious, and dealing with the darkness and inertness of depression can be anxiety provoking. Those with bipolar disorder tend to swing back and forth between high-energy, manic phases and deep depression.

But here's the kicker: everyone struggles with their mental health. It's just a matter of degrees.

Although each year 1 in 5 adult Americans experience mental illness, and 1 in 20 will experience serious mental illness, the remaining 80 percent of the population isn't necessarily stuck on calm and happy. Our moods are not binary, like an on-off switch for a light, but more like lights on a dimmer switch. The light comes up and down, and it is not always clear who or what is in control.

You don't need to have an official diagnosis of anxiety or depression to deal with the feelings of anxiety or depression: you only need to be human. So wherever one is on the mental health spectrum, it is nice to know something objective about the most subjective and abstract of things: our moods.

Anxiety

"You've got to give me a minute, 'cause I'm way down in it, and I can't breathe so I can't speak,"
—from "Anxiety" by Jason Isbell

We all worry, right? So, when does the obligatory and natural fretting become a problem? Answer: when the symptoms are either persistent or excessive. It's a problem when it becomes a problem: when the symptoms—not the owner of the symptoms—seem to be in charge. If you've ever attended a summer outdoor event where things turned buggy, there can be a tipping point where the bug problem goes racing past pesky to a maniacal swarming that keeps you from enjoying or even remembering what exactly you came there to do. Unless the host starts offering Benadryl martinis and blood transfusions, you're outta there.

The fear response built into our factory settings may not be entirely pleasant, but it is functional. Our caveman days are over, so we don't need to be worried about being eaten by a bear or getting attacked by a neighboring tribe. But life is still stressful, and the physiology of fear—championed by adrenaline and other stress hormones—is designed to make us physically and mentally focused. You want to be amped up for your big job interview, the looming deadline, or for any emergency that arises, and yet the stress we feel should be proportional to the threat. If just going to work feels like you're landing on the beach on D-Day, something isn't right. And when the challenge or the threat goes away, so should the stress. Regrettably, the stressors of modern life seem to come very close together, stacked up like cars on the interstate, so there is little time for recovery.

The "anxiety disorders" category includes the following (including, according to the American Psychiatric Association, the estimated percent of US adults in any given year with this particular form of anxiety):

Phobias (9 to 15 Percent)

This is where certain things or situations produce so much anxiety that one fears them. Agoraphobia—the fear of feeling trapped or helpless, particularly in public spaces—is the most common, but there are many others, and a disproportionate number of them end up as an answer on *Jeopardy!*

Social Anxiety Disorder (7 percent)

This isn't about being shy or introverted. It involves having an intense fear of being humiliated or judged in a social situation. It's high school on steroids.

Panic Disorder (2 to 3 percent)

Intense physical symptoms of anxiety—chest pain, a fast and thumping heart, shortness of breath, nausea—arrive suddenly, out of the blue, without any clear or particular stimulus (unlike what happens with phobias).

Separation Anxiety (1 to 2 percent)

This deals with having intense fears about being separated from home or from someone close to you.

Generalized Anxiety Disorder (GAD) (2 percent)

People with GAD worry excessively about *everything*. Given the ubiquitous nature of "everything," GAD can be a lot more difficult to live with than something like acrophobia—the fear of heights—which can generally be avoided unless you're a crane operator or a Mount Everest porter. Although generalized anxiety is not the most common anxiety disorder, its symptoms are the most universal, so let's focus on GAD.

Signs and Symptoms
An Overwhelming, Perpetual State of Worry or Dread
Like the rain in Seattle, the worrying just never seems to end. And if it doesn't happen to be raining, you're busy scanning the horizon for storm clouds (catastrophizing). You tell yourself, "This is all going to simmer down after the kids are out of the house, or after I get a different job, or after I patch up things with the family." Yet these milestones come and go and the worrying never ends. You start to worry about your worrying, and all of this leaves you cranky and irritable.

You've Forgotten How to Vacation or Relax
When you do occasionally manage to peel yourself away from the rat race, it takes three or four days just to start enjoying yourself. That's why a weekend at the beach or the mountains or the cabin is no longer particularly refreshing.

Your Mental Focus Is out of Focus; Your Mind Feels Overwhelmed
Your mind is a tangle of scattered thoughts, jumping from one thing to another. You try to plan your way out of this mess, but every contemplated move is checkmated by some competing worry.

You Thirst for Certainty—but the World Is Parched
The COVID pandemic proved how anxiety-provoking uncertainty can be. When the future is uncertain (honestly, isn't it always?), our brains go to work and begin concocting various scenarios of how things might go. This allows one to make plans, but if you've got a reasonably creative brain, or one that leans toward doomsday scenarios (apocalyptic storylines now seem to dominate TV the way Westerns did in the 1950s), your anxieties pile up on themselves like compound interest.

Sleep Problems
Of course you can't sleep. You can't turn off your brain.

Triple Espresso Physical Symptoms

Most, if not all, of the physical symptoms of anxiety can be explained by an excess of adrenaline. You feel like you sucked down a bottle of "155-Hour Energy Drink," symptoms of which include chest pain, a racing heart, feeling short of breath, a lump in the throat, sweaty hands and dry mouth, a shaky feeling, tingling in the fingers, or feeling light-headed because you're hyperventilating. Because constant adrenaline is exhausting, you're tired all the time, and the hypervigilance it causes makes one feel physically keyed-up and tense. You're so tight that the last time you had a massage they had to start off with a crowbar and a drum of WD-40. Jaw clenching and teeth grinding are also common.

Treatments for Anxiety

Before concluding that one's symptoms are entirely due to anxiety, one should have a doctor check to make sure it isn't an overactive thyroid gland that's sending the body into overdrive. There are a few other medical conditions that can mimic anxiety—like a tumor that is producing adrenaline—but these are exceptionally rare and are usually associated with very high blood pressure.

Psychotherapy, or Cognitive Behavioral Therapy (CBT)

Here, a therapist, psychologist, or psychiatrist can help patients recognize and unwind the tangled web of thoughts, subconscious beliefs, prior experiences, and recurrent emotional loops that lead to uncontrolled symptoms. It teaches you to say to your brain, "I see where you're taking me, and I am not going there." Therapy can also help identify "the slide" that warns of a possible up-cycling of symptoms, so one can intervene early and prevent a bad spell.

Medications

Medications like selective serotonin reuptake inhibitors (SSRIs) or serotonin-norepinephrine reuptake inhibitors (SNRIs) are the mainstay of medical therapy for anxiety, even though they are more commonly thought of as antidepressants. There *are* antianxiety medications such as Xanax, Klonopin, Valium, or Ativan, but because of their addictive potential and sedating side effects, they're typically prescribed only for acute attacks or very focused situations, and not as an everyday medication. Drugs called "beta-blockers" can help with mild anxiety symptoms (you might have heard of a colleague taking one before a big presentation) and the drug buspirone works somewhat like Xanax et al., but with lower side effects and risk of dependency.

Stress Reduction and Relaxation Techniques

Stress reduction and relaxation techniques such as deep breathing aren't just some New Age hocus pocus (well maybe some are, but have you ever noticed how relaxed and mellowed-out New Age people are?). It might sound absurdly simple, but choosing to stay positive and finding a way to laugh at the clown car of life can be very helpful (unless, of course, you have coulrophobia—the fear of clowns—then for heaven's sake pick another mental image). Other stress reduction options include exercise as well as yoga and tai chi. Described as "meditation in motion," a group doing tai chi can easily be mistaken for a group of synchronized mimes.

Meditation

If you're not familiar with meditation, you might see it as some Eastern religious practice, and if you stick with it you'll be ordering a backyard Buddhist shrine from Lowe's (some assembly required). In reality, although meditation developed as a spiritual practice adopted by various religions (Christians call it "centering prayer"), it can also be entirely non-religious and is sometimes referred to as "mind training." Techniques vary, but the essence of it is to quiet the perpetual emcee of one's inner thoughts. There are different techniques to do that, and they commonly include either focusing on a mantra—a word or sound that is repeated to calmly bring one back to center—or using a number of different meditative breathing practices as a calm and centering force.

Metaphors for meditation abound, but I like to think of it this way: rather than swimming in or paddling through the swift river of your thoughts and emotions, meditation has you sitting high up on the bank. From there, without comment or judgment, you just let…the river… flow…by. It's there in that quiet space, where the Me has finally been bound and gagged, that God or the Endless Void can get a wordless word in. If you're an atheist, think of it as hiring a dumpster for the mind, where you can dispose of all the crap that has piled up in the basement of your brain.

There is plenty of research proving how restorative and rejuvenating meditation can be. Like sleep, meditation seems to have a litany of physical benefits that go beyond improved brain health. Don't take it from me. Take it from comedian Jerry Seinfeld, a lifelong meditator, who said this on *Good Morning America* in 2021: "You know how your phone has a charger? [Meditation is] like if you had a charger for your whole body and mind, that's what [transcendental meditation] is."

Depression

> And you could have it all /
> My empire of dirt / I will let you down /
> I will make you hurt
> —*Nine Inch Nails, "Hurt"*

Although anxiety is more than twice as common as depression, it is depression that is the leading cause of disability worldwide. As with anxiety, depression is an excess of what are otherwise normal—if unpleasant—emotions. Hey, we all get gloomy, worried, unmotivated. Sometimes the gift of life seems more like the ashtray-flavored popcorn balls that my chain-smoking neighbors made for my siblings and me each and every Halloween. It's when negative feelings persist and become intense and excessive that problems begin.

Common Symptoms of Depression

- Feeling sad or having a depressed mood, most of the day, nearly every day
- Loss of interest or pleasure in the things you used to really enjoy—your favorite movie, food, or activity

- Problems with thinking or concentrating, feeling indecisive
- Loss of energy, increased fatigue
- Sleep problems: either too much or too little
- Feeling worthless, hopeless, or guilty
- Physical aches and pains (yes, how we're feeling physically is directly connected to how we're feeling emotionally)
- Changing appetite—weight gain or loss, without intentional change in diet
- Thoughts of being better off dead

Symptom checklists like these can be helpful, but it is worth noting that some people who experience depression describe a very particular *nothing*. They feel like someone turned their brain off, or that some cosmic force is pressing down on their soul. There is an emptiness of thought, motivation, and feeling that can be hard to describe.

Sadness vs. Depression

Depression is a lot more than what we felt like when the dog died, when there's trouble at work, or when we're having everyday relationship problems. Those things can certainly cause sadness, but sadness is different from depression. Sadness (and grief, too) is typically associated with a clear trigger, and doesn't drain life of all its joy. It can bring on regrets but not the hopelessness or worthlessness that can come with depression (i.e., with sadness you get to keep your self-esteem). Sadness is a glancing blow, a time-limited emotional stumble, compared to depression's prolonged feeling of having fallen into a deep, dark hole.

There are some simple depression screening tools on the Internet that will help you figure out where you are. Many of these are based on *The Diagnostic and Statistical Manual of Mental Disorders-5 (DSM-5-TR)*. It's a reference book published by the American Psychiatric Association that lists the diagnostic criteria for each and every mental health diagnosis, and it's available at the bookstore or library.

Causes of Depression

It's not clear what causes depression. Mood disorders like depression tend to run in families, so it may be an inherited alteration in brain biochemistry. The American Psychiatric Association notes that people who are generally pessimistic are more likely to experience depression, which calls to mind my Scandinavian heritage and the penchant for rationing positive emotions (always good to have some in reserve, in case you need them) and for staying happy by setting very low expectations ("It could be worse" is a well-recognized mantra here in Scandihoovian-leaning Minnesota).

Depression could be a learned behavior in the sense that one might adopt some of the behaviors of a depressed parent or sibling, for instance. It's clear that traumatic events, particularly as a child, can rewire the brain's emotional centers in a way that makes depression a recurrent issue. Prolonged psychosocial stress can trigger it, as can insomnia or drug abuse. Twenty-one percent of adults with substance abuse deal with depression, raising chicken-or-egg arguments about which came first.

Treatments for Depression

Before starting treatment, it's important to make sure there's no medical explanation for the symptoms, like a sleep disorder, a drug side effect, or an underactive thyroid—which has the effect of turning the idle on the body's engine way, way down.

Psychotherapy, or Cognitive Behavioral Therapy

As with anxiety, psychotherapy (talk therapy, cognitive behavioral therapy) can be very effective in untangling the web of thoughts, experiences, and emotions that lead to negative thinking.

Medications

Given how common anxiety and depression are, it's no wonder that SSRIs with trade names like Prozac, Paxil, Celexa, Zoloft, and Lexapro are now household names. These are not "happy pills" that will have you walking on water. But by putting one's brain chemistry into a healthier balance, they can be the life jacket that keeps one's head above water, allowing one to breathe and then marshal the resources and behaviors needed to climb back into the boat and join the party. SSRIs are not habit-forming. They can take several weeks or several months to fully kick in, and most psychiatrists recommend taking them for six months or more after the symptoms have improved. Some people will take them for life.

It'd be nice and *very convenient* if one could just take a pill and be fine. Maybe that's true for some people. But in most cases, although medications will improve symptoms, you'll have to do some soul and psyche work to really regain and restore your mental health.

ECT and TMS

Electroconvulsive therapy (ECT), aka "shock therapy," uses electricity to put the brain into a brief seizure, thereby reshuffling the mood deck in a way that we still don't particularly understand. But it does work, and ECT remains an option when rigorous use of therapy and medication has not been effective. Although the Frankenstein ghoulishness of ECT has faded with newer, much more technically sophisticated methods (prior to good muscle relaxants, the patient had to be strapped down to avoid flopping off the table), memory loss remains a possible side effect.

Transcranial magnetic stimulation (TMS) feels like a late model version of ECT. Electromagnetic pulses are delivered into the brain and are thought to activate and revive the nerves in the mood control center.

Exercise, Etc.

Yes, here we are again, talking about the mind benefits of physical activity! (In the high-pitched, critic-in-the-crowd voice of Jim Gaffigan: "He's talking about exercise *again*? All this talk about exercise is *exhausting* me. I need a nap!") But it's the truth: clinical studies show that for those with mild to moderate depression, regular aerobic exercise is as effective as antidepressants. In some countries it's even considered first-line therapy. A trip to the gym can be as good as a trip to the pharmacy—or better, given the litany of physical benefits that come with exercise.

A non-pharmacological therapy option for those wintering in higher latitudes (Scandinavians!) is light therapy. There's some science supporting us when we describe someone as having a "sunny disposition."

Suicide

On the face of it, a person with paranoid schizophrenia might be considered to have a "serious mental illness," whereas someone with depression might be thought of as having something less serious. But that ignores the reality that depression can be a lethal illness, primarily via suicide.

In the United States, suicide rates have increased 35 percent since 1999, and you've undoubtedly heard the troubling news about declining US life expectancy due to an increase in mortality rates for adults ages 25 to 64. Although initial data suggested the trend was only in white men, follow-up data showed increases across all age groups and both sexes, and that the deaths were largely due to suicide, poisonings (opioid and alcohol overdosing), and chronic liver disease due to alcoholism. The largest increases were noted in the Ohio Valley and New England, leading to speculation that these were "deaths of despair," caused by the realization of many that they will be less well-off than their parents, and that for them the new economy means financial hardship—overwhelming college debt and/or an economy with fewer good-paying blue-collar jobs leaving them behind.

Risk Factors and Warning Signs

Almost half of the people who die by suicide *do not* have a known mental health condition, so worrisome symptoms and behaviors are a better indicator of risk than any mental health diagnoses. Here's what to watch out for.

Subtle Early Warning Signs
The clues can start small, with comments like "I'd be better off gone," "I feel stuck," or "This is hopeless," little quips that sound off-hand enough to make it difficult to know how serious the person is being. It can be awkward to ask, but a simple clarifying question like "What do you mean by that?" can be a good start. *Let's be clear: asking someone if they are having suicidal thoughts will not put that idea in their head!* Asking hard questions, even if you have to stumble through the words, shows that you care, and that itself could save someone's life.

Not-So-Subtle Warning Signs

There are certain behaviors that signal things are really cycling down: withdrawing from friends and family; dropping activities that used to really be their "thing"; increasingly impulsive, reckless, angry, or aggressive behavior; dramatic mood swings; increasing alcohol or drug use.

Warning Signs Give Way to Worrisome Behaviors

These behaviors suggest a person is moving close to the edge, and it's time to get serious and intervene: saying their goodbyes to friends and family, tying up loose personal or financial ends, or saving pills so that one can overdose. And for people who live where hunting and guns aren't a common part of life, another warning sign could be buying a weapon.

Speaking of guns, a few years ago I lost a childhood friend to suicide by firearm. He struggled mightily with depression for many years; toward the end, he was cycling down. Suicide was a serious concern and was discussed openly. He was not a "gun freak" or part of a militia, but he had a lot of guns, and they were important to him. Taking them all away, even if that were possible, also seemed to run the risk of deepening his depression. It was a very difficult situation, and certainly not unique to him.

Risk Factors for Suicide

Serious Relationship problems: Per the CDC, this is the top factor contributing to suicide.

Gender: Women attempt suicide more often than men, but men are three to four times as likely to die in the attempt.

Alcohol: One in three people who die from suicide are intoxicated. For someone in my line of work, the perpetually festive beer ads on TV are a cruel satire.

A family history of suicide: Maybe it's genetic, but perhaps having a family history of suicide makes this final act of despair feel more like an option, and not an entirely unthinkable act.

Access to firearms: It's the most common method of suicide (about half of cases).

Age: Older adults are more likely to attempt suicide, and more likely to be "successful" at it.

A recent loss: Such as an academic or business failure, financial or legal issues.

Prolonged stress, a serious or chronic medical illness, a history of abuse or trauma: Combat vets are an unfortunately common example.

What to Do in a Suicide Crisis: Remain Calm, Empathize, Forge a Mutual Plan

If you are trying to help someone who's in a suicide crisis, you will certainly not feel settled on the inside. Despite this, aim to project a sense of calm with Oscar-winning authority. Fear, panic, and anxiety are highly contagious and spread telepathically.

Calmly clarify their intentions:

- Did you hear them right?
- How serious are they—do they have a plan?
- Have they already taken an overdose—if so, what and when?

Calmly suggest a mutual plan:

- "Let's call your psychiatrist."
- "Let's call a mental health hotline and see if they can help us."
- "Let's get this checked out at the ER."

Calmly call for backup from friends and family.

Though you might well be angry, outraged, or confused, put a cork in all that and convey empathy—how difficult it must be for them to feel this low, how sad you are for them in this moment. You can have a lively debate about the moral, psychological, financial, and familial implications of suicide later.

The Shame of It, the Blame of It

Mental health stands apart from physical health in three ways:

1. The diagnosis of mental health conditions is almost entirely subjective. Blood tests can tell if you're anemic—to what degree, and probably even why you're low on blood. But there's no "karma quotient" or "delusional level" that we can measure. Brain MRIs don't tell us anything. So patients and mental health providers are left searching for the words to describe what's going on inside a patient's head and in their soul, and that can be a difficult task.
2. Some medical issues—high blood pressure, diabetes, obesity—are common, but they are not universal. Conversely, working to maintain one's own mental health balance is a ubiquitous, omnipresent task, a part of being human. People can (and most, if not all, do) struggle with symptoms of anxiety or depression without having a full-fledged disorder. Even delusional thinking—a false, fixed belief that is held despite evidence to the contrary—is more widespread than one might think, occurring on a spectrum from pesky to dysfunctional to severely disabling in a schizophrenic patient.
3. Then there's the shame of having mental health issues. People can and do talk openly about their diabetes, kidney stones, or heart disease. Who hasn't listened to someone's backyard barbecue soliloquy on the twists and turns of their last bout of diverticulitis? But when the topic turns to anxiety, depression, or a friend's struggles with a schizophrenic adult son—these things come in whispers and hints. A public panic attack warrants, all too often, a shaming. Have you watched Ted Lasso?

Suicide has shame in spades. I know from experience that survivors are often hobbled by guilt: "Wasn't there more that we could have done?" Obituaries for those who ended their own life often speak in code, saying that the deceased "died at home after struggling with a chronic illness." This is the truth, but only part of it, and so the shame lives on.

Not only does shame keep mental health issues out of the public view; it also keeps it bottled up inside sufferers, a very private war. The majority of those who have died by suicide had not expressed their intentions to anyone. One would think that that much despair, under that kind of pressure, would have to leak out, but somehow those who suffer so manage to keep it all in.

No one says this out loud, but there's still this idea floating around in our subconscious that mental health disorders only happen to the weak-minded. Recommending (even with the best of intentions) that someone who is depressed just "pull themselves up by their bootstraps" is a blame game that we don't play with physical health problems. We would never say, "I guess she's got kidney issues. I bet if she just put on her big-girl panties, she could get rid of half of her pills."

Depression Is an Illness, Not a Weakness
—Blog title, National Alliance on
Mental Illness (nami.org)

Mental Health Hygiene

After you've oiled and reinforced your bootstraps, here are some additional ways you can optimize your mental health. If you've read through a list like this before, you'll note that mental health tips often have a back-to-basics theme. Life was never simple, but its increasing complexity and frenetic pace has pulled us away from the things that really satisfy and refresh our souls. So back we go.

Mindfulness

The point is that you have one. You have a mind with thoughts, emotions, worries, and fears, and ignoring all of that is not a useful management strategy. If the house turns chilly, you don't just "tough it out." You fiddle with the thermostat. You grab a hoodie. You adjust. Pay attention to your mind.

Time Out!

The American approach to winning at life is to grab it by the throat and choke the daylights out of it. Work harder, faster. Do more. Achieve. And when you do finally decide to tackle your depression, it will be an all-out blitz of therapy sessions, mental health podcasts, medications, support groups. Instead, we need to relax. Slow down. Turn your brain off (via meditation). Stick close to friends and family, but turn the rest of the world off. Leave your AirPods at home when you go for a walk or run. Resist the urge to be perpetually entertained. Leave enough space so that you can hear yourself think. Rather than attacking your problems with a closed fist, try an open hand.

Stay in the Moment

It sounds like a country song or a Hallmark card, but it's absolutely true: yesterday is in the past, and tomorrow hasn't yet arrived. Avoiding deep forays into the future is one way to stop catastrophizing.

Positive Attitude and Gratitude

Scientifically proven! No, a painted-on cheerleader smile is not going to dissolve your problems away like honey in your tea, but attitude matters. Seeing the glass as half full rather than half empty is a matter of gratitude: it's a conscious decision to recognize what has been received (half a glass of water) rather than what has been taken away.

Exercise

The mind-body connection is real. The days that you *absolutely* don't have time to go for a walk, are *exactly* the days that you will most benefit from going for a walk.

Sleep

Nothing good comes from poor sleep. It's hard to overestimate sleep deprivation's contribution to our rising mental health woes. Maybe that's because sleep is when the mental dumpster gets emptied.

Burn Good Fuel

Healthy food is healthy fuel. Sugars in particular, like the shovelful dissolved in your frappuccino, tend to just pump you up and dump you down.

Meditation

See anxiety section. For a good reboot, put the phone down and turn off your brain at regular intervals.

Seek Community

Humans are tribal. It's not just that we naturally clump together, it's that other people are therapy. They're good medicine. They help us make sense of our lives. They commiserate. This doesn't mean that an introvert needs to be the life of the party, grabbing the mic at the karaoke stage. They just need to be there, in back with the others, making fun of the tone-deaf extroverts up on the stage. People living in strong social networks live better and longer.

What about Social Media?

When it comes to mental health hygiene, is social media a ray of sunshine that allows us to make and maintain the strong social connections we know can help us stay balanced and resilient? Or is it more like a parasite, sucking the life force out of us? Polling shows that many find social media to be anxiety-provoking, depressing, and caustic to one's self-esteem. We easily recognize these four components of digital stress:

- The fear of missing out (FOMO)
- Communication overload (too many notifications)
- Availability stress (it's on all the time, but should I be?)
- Approval anxiety (monitoring for likes and affirming comments; catastrophizing over a text message that received no reply)

Scientists who study the interplay of social media and mental health describe it as nuanced and complicated, primarily because there are so many independent variables. Every user has his or her own unique psychological profile, with different levels of self-esteem and propensities for anxiety or depression. Does a user have a strong offline social support network, or is Facebook their family? At what level does one engage with social media—not just how often, but to what degree (are you just a "liker" or do you make comments or post content)?

Is social media sunshine on your shoulders, or worms in your stool? You decide.

YOU'RE GOING TO LIVE FOREVER

And I'm Going to Learn How to Fly. Theories on Aging.

H umans have been searching for the fountain of youth as long as we've been dying. So far, we have little to show for our efforts.

Juan Ponce de León went looking for it in Florida. It didn't have the fountain he was looking for, but it did have 30,000 acres that would one day become home to the Magic Kingdom and the powerful Disney empire. Ironically, León's quest for eternal youth ended in his premature death. On a return trip to the Sunshine State, he was shot with a poison arrow by native Floridians who apparently weren't interested in being discovered.

What we do understand about the fountain of youth is that the drain plug works pretty well for a few years, cradling our aqua splendor, but eventually it begins a slow leak sometime in the third decade of life.

There are many theories on why we age, on why the fountain goes dry, but the science of aging revolves around two basic ideas:

MAN OVERBOARD!

Immortality remains evasive. Aging is either a genetically programmed fuse (could telomeres be that fuse?) or a series of inevitable mistakes and injuries that add up over time.

1. Human life is of a genetically preprogrammed duration.
2. Aging and death are the culmination of a series of unplanned errors (a "shit happens" kind of view).

Programmed Cell Death: Your Days Are Numbered, and Your Genes Are Doing the Counting

The "programmed theory" sees aging as inevitable: the spring on the alarm clock can be wound up once, and when that stored energy is fully released, the clock stops. There is a strong genetic component to this theory of aging, and it may be most famously represented by the work of Leonard Hayflick, a scientist who noted that most cells can divide only a finite number of times.

This limit is thought to be a function of telomeres, the plastic cap on the end of our genetic (chromosome) shoelaces that gets a little shorter every time the cell divides and our chromosomes need to be duplicated. When the telomere cap is gone, the chromosomal shoelace begins to fray. Thereafter, the cell either implodes and dies (apoptosis), or it goes into a neutral "senescent" stage—alive and still communicating and interacting with its communal cellular neighbors, but no longer able to divide. Been there, done that.

One common example of this programmed theory of aging would be the appearance of gray hair. The pigment-producing portion of a hair follicle goes through a certain number of repetitions of making pigment, and then it just up and quits: thereafter, the hair turns gray or white due to lack of pigment. Is this explanation at odds with the common claim that it's children that give their parents gray hair? Not necessarily. The study of epigenetics suggests that our physical, chemical, and even psychosocial environments can change the way our genes are expressed, turning some on and some off. It is therefore entirely possible, even likely, that the stress of repeatedly dealing with your standard incredulous hormone-soaked teenager could cause the genes in the hair follicle pigment cells to be turned off prematurely, turning gray with exasperation.

Mistakes Have Been Made—the Error Theory

The second major category of aging theories is called the "Error Theory." This theory says that genetic blueprints don't call for us to wear out and die, at least not this early, but mistakes have been made, and mistakes add up.

The human genome consists of 23 pairs of chromosomes containing approximately 30,000 genes made up of about 3 billion base pairs of DNA, so the potential for error is real. Not every genetic mutation is necessarily bad ("Look, Ma! My thumbs are opposable!"), nor is it even expressed. Singular events that change the world are interesting and dramatic (Lee Harvey Oswald's almost unbelievable ballistic luck, for instance), but major changes usually come about as a result of a collection of smaller events. World War II, for example, wasn't won with a single bullet or with a single battle.

The Error Catastrophe Theory of aging speaks to this idea, stating that smaller genetic and/or metabolic mistakes, perhaps inconsequential on an individual basis, add up over time and eventually lead to something catastrophic for an individual cell.

In 2007, a major interstate bridge in downtown Minneapolis suddenly collapsed during rush hour, killing 13 people and injuring 145 more. It collapsed in an instant, but it took a long time to get to that instant. It wasn't one weak bolt or gusset plate that did it in. It was a series of slow, chronic failures and miscalculations that led to the very sudden, acute failure.

Gene replication is, in essence, a transmission of information—every new cell must have an owner's manual. But like the now ancient game of Telephone, where a message is whispered person-to-person down a long line, small errors made early on in the process can eventually become compounded, so that when the message finally gets to the end of the line, Neville Chamberlain's "I believe it is peace for our time," becomes "Ivy League geese chimes."

Although some of these genetic errors occur during cell division, some happen when the cell is just sitting around doing its cellular thing.

The Free Radical Theory is one of the leading ideas in the "Error Theory" category. We humans are continually doing a slow burn: we burn our food using oxygen, but we do it slowly enough to avoid any flames. Inside the cell, an organelle called a mitochondrion serves as the energy plant of the cell. Most of the time the burn is fairly clean (picture a nice bed of orange coals), but sometimes the burning process is less efficient (picture a smoldering smoky fire). Inefficient oxidation can produce free radicals—oddly charged atoms and molecules that are chemically unstable. These free radicals bounce around cells and abrade and damage whatever it is they strike. If a free radical gets into the nucleus of the cell where the DNA is stored, mutations can occur. There's some evidence to suggest that old mitochondria become less efficient, thereby producing more free radicals.

The "Error Theory" category also includes the Wear-and-Tear Theory, which suggests that the more you *use*, the more you *lose*. That fits with the fact that animals with high metabolic rates tend to live the shortest lives, and those with the lowest metabolic rates tend to live the longest.

Mammals, for instance, get about a billion heartbeats in a lifetime.

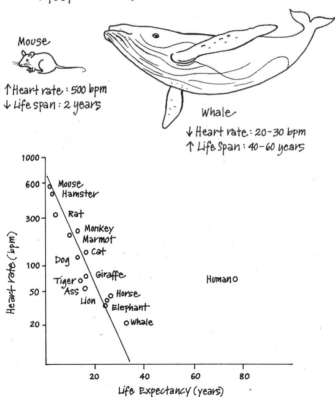

MAN OVERBOARD!

The mouse in your garage, with a blistering-fast heart rate, uses them up quickly and has a short lifespan. The dog on your couch, with a heart rate around 100 beats per minute, uses them up a little more slowly. Gray whales, with a heart rate in the mid-30's when surfacing and far lower than that when diving, use them up very slowly, and have a life expectancy that may reach into the 70s.

Humans buck those trends. We far outlive animals like the tiger that have a similar heart rate as ours (60 to 90 beats per minute) but typically die as teenagers. What is it that allows us to outlive our fellow mammals, to get closer to 2.5 billion heartbeats in a lifetime?

It's easy to attribute our longevity to the conveniences of modern life: health care, nutrition, and sanitation. But humans were long-lived even before life got modern—even if life expectancy data suggests otherwise. Remember, life expectancy really means "life expectancy at birth," so the death of an infant or a childbearing mother (a very common event back in the day) heavily skewed life expectancy data. Life expectancy in the United States in 1900 was around 47 years, but there were plenty of people who lived far longer than that—if they could make it through the highly mortal gauntlet of birth, infancy, and childbirth. If we're honest, basic sanitation has done far more for human life expectancy than coronary angioplasty has.

Without getting too complicated or sciency, let's just say that the unique longevity of our species is due to "the magic sauce." But eventually, even the magic runs out. What I call "The Graph of Impending Death" and what aging staticians and actuarials call the "WTF! Graph" looks a bit like a checkmark. The chance of dying starts out high at infancy but falls quickly. It begins rising in the teen years, levels off briefly in our twenties and early thirties, and after age 40 rises steadily toward the afterlife.

If you're looking to never die, may I suggest getting extensions for your telomeres, or cryopreservation? If you're looking to flatten out your own personal WTF! Graph, take a look at the work of Dan Buettner. He's spent his career studying the world's longest-lived people in five different geographic pockets—what he termed Blue Zones—and found a number of commonalities. They live active, high-NEAT lives, have strong ties with family and friends, and belong to a faith-based community. They are careful not to overeat and have diets rich in beans and low in meat. They de-stress with a nap, a prayer, or happy hour with friends. They like a glass of wine with friends or a meal. It's that simple, and it's that complicated.

No doubt there are some good genes and good luck involved, but it's worth noting that the centenarians Buettner chronicles have lived *well*, not just long.

I've had the honor of caring for hundreds of patients who've lived into their nineties and hundreds. I routinely ask them for the secret to their longevity, and they routinely reply, with a gratitude-imbued chuckle, "Oh, I don't know…" As far as I can tell, they unwittingly spent their lives in their own little Blue Zone, so that was a big help. But I'll add one thing to Buettner's list: these people love to laugh. If my clinical experience has taught me anything, it's hard to make it into your nineties without a sense of humor. All the crabasses are dead by then. Don't be one of them.

"There's a big old goofy man
dancing with a big old goofy girl,
Ooh baby, it's a big old goofy world"
—*John Prine, "It's a Big Old Goofy World"*

ACKNOWLEDGMENTS

The entire staff at Mayo Clinic Press, including Daniela Rapp and Dan Simmons. For letting me be me, within reason.

Jennifer Thompson, Isabelle Bleecker, and Nathan Vogt at Nordlyset Literary Agency. Thanks for finding me (that's not how it's supposed to work), and for listening to Wendy.

Steph. For your love, and for the time away—even when there didn't seem to be any. For encouraging me in this concoctive craft, and for being the "first eyes" on everything. And for explaining to the kids that 'Your dad has a problem: he's a writer.'

Julia. Isak. Caleb. Each of you were my favorite child. Keep that to yourself. I love you.

Clarice. For giving me the love of words—either in my genes, or through your faithful letters, or by reading the magical books of L. Frank Baum to us. In another time, I would have had to share you with a trove of university students.

Denis Lyman. You made me laugh. Still do. Your cynicism about the overeducated follows me and keeps me grounded. There wasn't a person in this world you couldn't and wouldn't talk to. I hated it as a kid, but I was listening. Let's go fishing.

Nancy Louise. I inherited your nose for details, which is probably why I became an internist. Sorry I used some swear words. You're a great mom. I love you.

At Augustana College (IL): Karin Youngberg. For the sit-down freshman year, informing me—in no uncertain terms—that I was really an English major masquerading as a Pre-Med major. Don Erickson, Ann Boaden, and Roald Tweet: for accepting me as an apprentice in the writer's guild.

Laurel. For single-handedly elevating my status in the residency draft. For being a colleague, friend, confidante, "second eyes" editor, provider of manure and honey, and for channeling the spirit of Ms. Efteland.

Claus. For showing me that art—and the joy it brings—is *everywhere*.

Steve Kaplan. You took me to lunch and told me you couldn't give me a writing gig, but knew people who could, and should.

Jeff Johnson. You "got" my writing instantly and gave me a monthly column. I twirled around the MTM statue on Nicollet Mall afterward. You made writing *so much fun*.

Ron Glasser. You were a physician writing at the highest level and thought I could too. You gave me names to call and a kick in the shorts.

Terry, Claus, Laurel, Ed, and Hallie. For teaching me how to think, and how to care for patients.

Kerri Miller and Michael Osterholm. For your mastery of explaining complicated concepts with clarity and imagination (you set a high bar). And for the gift of affirmation.

To my medical content reviewers, with deep gratitude. Joe Jensen, Mike Miedema, Brian Swiglo, David Ingham, John Seng, Tim Sullivan, Scott Sharkey, Linda Brady, Jonathan Hovda, Kevin Grullon, Ensor Transfeldt, Mary Beth Lardizabal, Ron Shapiro, John Lesser.

To the early adapters. Loren, Claus and Rose, Carleton, Peter B, Peter M, Jeff and Dianne, Ron and Judy, Bob, Ed and Donna, John C., Lynn, Jon and Jenny, Dick, George, Hannah and Steve, Bob and Judy, Mary Spazzicola, Jake and Karen, Mary and Kevin, and Darrin and Diana.

For personal professional support. Tim Madigan, Chris Dall, Tim Sullivan, Jason Peters, Kent Krueger, Susan Albright, Emily Gurnon.

David Tierney. For your creative juices, enthusiasm, and technical wizardry.

Bruce Cockburn. Finding your music in high school changed how I saw the world. Your songs were (and remain) transportive, your lyrics Jedi.

Wendell Berry. You are the Smartest Person in the Universe. Your works will endure. I continue to be deeply honored—and also guilt-stricken—that you've wasted time and postage on me.

ENDNOTES

I set out to make *Man Overboard!* a fun-to-read handbook for health, rather than a not-fun-to-read academic textbook. I wanted to be sure to make the big things the big things, so I focused on The Rules, rather than The Exceptions to the Rules (which typically foster controversy rather than clarity).

With that in mind, I've generally avoided talking in great detail about this specific study, or that particular research article; but if I did, I cited the information below using a "blind endnote" style. It starts with an italicized snippet of the text being referred to, followed by the source. (*Four score and seven years ago*: Abraham Lincoln, "Gettysburg Address," Journal of Unprecedented Carnage and Dismemberment, November 19, 1863.)

Much of what I had to say is an amalgamation of years of education and professional experience and is not directly attributable to one particular source. Given the general nature of *Man Overboard!*, many of the details I've gathered together are widely available from a variety of different sources. Nevertheless, I include some of the articles, websites, or books that I drew inspiration and/or information from. A few might be too technical or detailed for readers to find interesting, but many are very accessible and will give you a sense of where I've been, and where you can go too.

If this is all more than you care to look at, you can jump to the end, where I've included a short list of what I consider to be bedrock health information resources.

Prologue
Laughter is immeasurable: Wendell Berry, from the poem "Manifesto: The Mad Farmer Liberation Front"

Andropause
they shelled out $300 million: Spending for DTC Advertising and Detailing to Health Care Professionals 2008, Congressional Budget Office, https://www.cbo.gov/sites/default/files/111th-con-

gress-2009-2010/reports/12-02-drugpromo_brief.pdf

Unfortunately, this heady epoch: Katherine Ellen Foley, "Pfizer is releasing its own generic Viagra to stay relevant," Quartz, Dec. 6, 2017, https://qz.com/1149322/pfizer-is-releasing-a-generic-viagra-as-its-patent-expires/

In all fairness, these marketeers: Stuart Elliot, "Viagra and the Battle of the Awkward Ads," *New York Times*, April 25, 2004. https://www.nytimes.com/2004/04/25/business/viagra-and-the-battle-of-the-awkward-ads.html

And though he could have easily driven around it: Pfizer Viagra ad, "This Is the Age of Taking Action," https://www.ispot.tv/ad/7kNk/viagra-the-age-of-knowing-how-to-make-things-happen

The quiz seems more like: John E. Morley et al., "Validation of a screening questionnaire for androgen deficiency in aging males," *Metabolism*, Sept. 1, 2000, Vol 49. https://www.metabolismjournal.com/article/S0026-0495(00)25964-7/pdf#relatedArticles

"The prevalence of even the most specific": Frederick Wu et al., "Identification of Late-Onset Hypogonadism in Middle-Aged and Elderly Men," *New England Journal of Medicine*, July 8, 2010, https://www.nejm.org/doi/pdf/10.1056/NEJMoa0911101

...the prestigious Institute of Medicine completed a systematic review: "Testosterone and Aging: Clinical Research Directions," Institute of Medicine (US) Committee on Assessing the Need for Clinical Trials of Testosterone Replacement Therapy https://pubmed.ncbi.nlm.nih.gov/25009850/

Here's what they found: Snyder et al., "Lessons from the Testosterone Trials," *Endocrine Reviews*, 2018 Jun 1; 39(3):369-386, https://pubmed.ncbi.nlm.nih.gov/29522088/

American College of Physicians performed a sweeping review: Amir Qaseem et al. "Testosterone treatment in adult men with age-related low testosterone: A clinical guideline from the American College of Physicians," *Ann Intern Med*, Jan 2020. https://www.acpjournals.org/doi/pdf/10.7326/M19-0882

Testosterone Tales

The female sex chromosome has 1,090 genes: Daniel Federman, "The Biology of Human Sex Differences," *New England Journal of Medicine*, April 2006; 354:1507-14, https://www.nejm.org/doi/pdf/10.1056/NEJMra052529

twice the mutation frequency: ibid

What the bumbling, fumbling male sex: "SRY Gene," National Library of Medicine, MedlinePlus, https://medlineplus.gov/genetics/gene/sry/

The testes actually secrete three: John Hall, Guyton and Hall *Textbook of Medical Physiology 13th edition.* https://www.amazon.com/Guyton-Hall-Textbook-Medical-Physiology/dp/1455770051

"sex hormone binding globulin": David Handelsman, "Androgen Physiology, Pharmacology, Use and Misuse," *Endotext*, Oct 5, 2020, https://www.ncbi.nlm.nih.gov/books/NBK279000/

trigger the release of testosterone: Anna Goldman et. al, "A Reappraisal of Testosterone's Binding in Circulation: Physiological and Clinical Implications," *Endocrine Reviews*, Aug. 2017, https://pubmed.ncbi.nlm.nih.gov/28673039/

The largest fraction of a man's estrogen levels: John Hall, Guyton and Hall *Textbook of Medical Physiology 13th edition.* https://www.amazon.com/Guyton-Hall-Textbook-Medical-Physiology/dp/1455770051

The testes make 7000 ug of testosterone: "The Biology of Human Sex Differences Federman, *New England Journal of Medicine*, April 2006; 354:1507-14 https://www.nejm.org/doi/pdf/10.1056/NEJMra052529

"Thus, each tissue can construct its own": Ibid

50% more muscle mass: John Hall, Guyton and Hall *Textbook of Medical Physiology 13th edition.* https://www.amazon.com/Guyton-Hall-Textbook-Medical-Physiology/dp/1455770051

Visible enough to detect on MRI scans: Rebecca Knickmeyer et al., "Impact of Sex and Gonadal Steroids on Neonatal Brain Structure," *Cerebral Cortex*, 2013, https://pubmed.ncbi.nlm.nih.gov/23689636/

men are more likely: Ibid

women's superior linguistic skills: Dardo Tomasi and Nora Volkow, "Laterality Patterns of Brain Functional Connectivity: Gender Effects," *Cerebral Cortex*, June 2012, https://pubmed.ncbi.nlm.nih.gov/21878483/

old and fading theory of sexual brain development: Margaret McCarthy and Arthur Arnold, "Reframing Sexual Differentiation of the Brain," *Nat Neuroscience*, June 2011, https://pubmed.ncbi.nlm.nih.gov/21613996/

Given how actively our brains interact: Eric Keverne et al., "Epigenetic changes in the developing brain: Effects on Behavior," *PNAS*, June 2015, https://www.pnas.org/doi/10.1073/pnas.1501482112

Great Sexpectations
Kevin McVary, "Erectile Dysfunction," *New England Journal of Medicine*, 2007; 357: 2472-2481 https://www.nejm.org/doi/full/10.1056/NEJMcp067261

National Social Life, Health and Aging Project (NSHAP): Stacy Lindau et al., "A Study of Sexuality and Health Among Older Adults in the United States," *New England Journal of Medicine*, Aug 23, 2007. Table 2, Table 4, https://www.nejm.org/doi/full/10.1056/NEJMoa067423

"International Index of Erectile Function" quiz: https://www.baus.org.uk/_userfiles/pages/files/Patients/Leaflets/iief.pdf

"Sexual Inventory for Men" (SHIM): https://www.pfizerpro.com/sites/default/files/shim_vgu610709-01.pdf

In the late 1980's and early 1990's, researchers at Pfizer: Ian Osterloh, "How I Discovered Viagra," *Cosmos*, April 27, 2015 https://cosmosmagazine.com/science/biology/how-i-discovered-viagra/

A review of 14 trials: Howard Fink et al., "Sildenafil for Male Erectile Dysfunction: A systematic review and meta-analysis," *JAMA Internal Medicine*, June 24, 2002 https://jamanetwork.com/journals/jamainternalmedicine/fullarticle/211714

Another study took 123 men: Artur Carvalho et al.,"The Management of Erectile Dysfunction with Placebo Only: Does it Work?," *Journal of Sexual Medicine*, Dec 1, 2009 https://www.jsm.jsexmed.org/article/S1743-6095(15)32350-X/fulltext

Not to fear: priapism is a rare event: Florian Roghmann, "Incidence of Priapism in Emergency Departments in the United States," *J Urology*, Oct 2013. https://www.auajournals.org/doi/pdf/10.1016/j.juro.2013.03.118

Bald Is Beautiful, but Is It Unhealthy?
William Cranwell and Rodney Sinclair, "Male Androgenetic Alopecia," *Endotext*, Feb 29, 2016 https://www.ncbi.nlm.nih.gov/books/NBK278957/

The International Society of Hair Restoration Surgery https://ishrs.org/patients/treatments-for-hair-loss/

Vera Price, "Treatment of Hair Loss," *New England Journal of Medicine*, Sept 23, 1999. https://www.nejm.org/doi/10.1056/NEJM199909233411307

In 2013, researchers from Tokyo University: Tomohide Yamada et al., "Male Pattern Baldness and Its Association with Coronary Heart Disease: a meta-analysis," *BMJ Open*, 2013, https://bmjopen.bmj.com/content/bmjopen/3/4/e002537.full.pdf

One small study stands out: Gita Faghihi et al. "The effectiveness of adding low-level light therapy to minoxidil 5% solution in the treatment of patients with androgenetic alopecia," *Indian Journal of Dermatology, Venereology, and Leprology*, July 2018, https://ijdvl.com/the-effectiveness-of-adding-low-level-light-therapy-to-minoxidil-5-solution-in-the-treatment-of-patients-with-androgenetic-alopecia/

Low Back Pain
Roger Chou, "Low Back Pain," *Annals of Internal Medicine*, August 2021, https://www.acpjournals.org/doi/pdf/10.7326/AITC202108170

Richard Deyo and James Weinstein, "Low Back Pain," *New England Journal of Medicine*, Feb 1, 2001, https://www.nejm.org/doi/full/10.1056/NEJM200102013440508

Christian Ruff, "NSAIDS: How dangerous are they for your heart?" Heart Health, *Harvard Health Publishing* https://www.health.harvard.edu/blog/nsaids-how-dangerous-are-they-for-your-heart-2019010715677

very difficult to tell what exactly is the source: Roger Chou et al., "Diagnosis and Treatment of Low Back Pain: A Joint Clinical Practice Guideline from the American College of Physicians and the American Pain Society," *Annals of Internal Medicine,* Oct. 2007, https://www.acpjournals.org/doi/full/10.7326/0003-4819-147-7-200710020-00006

In 2017, the American College of Physicians reviewed: Amir Qaseem et al., "Noninvasive Treatments for Acute, Subacute, and Chronic Low Back Pain: A Clinical Practice Guideline from the American College of Physicians," *Annals of Internal Medicine,* April 2017, https://www.acpjournals.org/doi/10.7326/M16-2367?_ga=2.125057485.677574257.1613447808-597910048.1613447808

Is spinal manipulation safe?: "Spinal Manipulation: What You Need to Know," National Center for Complementary and Integrative Health https://www.nccih.nih.gov/health/spinal-manipulation-what-you-need-to-know

CDC estimates that from 1999 to 2018: Drug Overdose Deaths, Prescription Opioids, CDC, https://www.cdc.gov/drugoverdose/deaths/prescription/overview.html

Fortunately, opioid prescribing rates: Drug Overdose Deaths, Prescribing Practices, Changes in Opioid Prescribing Practices, CDC. https://www.cdc.gov/drugoverdose/deaths/prescription/practices.html

Dr. Howard Schubiner succinctly summarizes: Juno DeMelo, "I Have to Believe This Book Cured My Pain," *New York Times,* Nov 9, 2021, https://www.nytimes.com/2021/11/09/well/mind/john-sarno-chronic-pain-relief.html

A 2009 review by the American Pain Society: Roger Chou et al., "Surgery for Low Back Pain: a review of the evidence for an American Pain Society Clinical Practice Guideline," *Spine,* May 1, 2009. https://pubmed.ncbi.nlm.nih.gov/19363455/

Vices

Smoking

Since the release of Dr. Terry's landmark report: "Health Consequences of Smoking, Surgeon General Fact Sheet," U.S. Department of Health and Human Services, https://www.hhs.gov/surgeongeneral/reports-and-publications/tobacco/consequences-smoking-factsheet/index.html

In 1988 the U.S. Consumer Product Safety Commission: Statement by Anne Graham, Commissioner, letter titled "Decision to Ban Lawn Darts," May 25, 1988. From "CPSC Votes Lawn Dart Ban," Consumer Products Safety Commission. https://www.cpsc.gov/Newsroom/News-Releases/1988/CPSC-Votes-Lawn-Dart-Ban

U.S. smoking rates from 21%: "Current Cigarette Smoking Among Adults in the United States," CDC, https://www.cdc.gov/tobacco/data_statistics/fact_sheets/adult_data/cig_smoking/index.htm

smoking rates remain highest in these groups: ibid

in late 2016 the FDA removed: "FDA Revises description of mental health side effects of the stop-smoking medicines Chantix (varenicline) and Zyban (bupropion) to reflect clinical trial findings," https://www.fda.gov/files/drugs/published/Drug-Safety-Communication--FDA-revises-description-of-mental-health-side-effects-of-the-stop-smoking-medicines-Chantix-%28varenicline%29-and-Zyban-%28bupropion%29-to-reflect-clinical-trial-findings-%28PDF%29.pdf

In 2016, a British study found: Nicola Lindson-Hawley et al., "Gradual Versus Abrupt Smoking Cessation," *Annals of Internal Medicine,* May 2016, https://www.acpjournals.org/doi/10.7326/M14-2805?articleid=2501853

The CDC's "bottom line": "Adult Smoking Cessation—The Use of E-Cigarettes," CDC, https://www.cdc.gov/tobacco/data_statistics/sgr/2020-smoking-cessation/fact-sheets/adult-smoking-cessation-e-cigarettes-use/index.html

A 2015 survey found: "Smoking Cessation: Fast Facts," CDC, https://www.cdc.gov/tobacco/data_statistics/fact_sheets/cessation/smoking-cessation-fast-facts/index.html

Alcohol
"Alcohol Use in the United States; Alcohol Facts and Statistics," *National Institute on Alcohol Abuse and Alcoholism*, https://www.niaaa.nih.gov/publications/brochures-and-fact-sheets/alcohol-facts-and-statistics
four subcategories of "excessive alcohol use": "Excessive Alcohol Use," National Center for Chronic Disease Prevention and Health Promotion, CDC, https://www.cdc.gov/chronicdisease/resources/publications/factsheets/alcohol.htm
what constitutes a drink: "What Is a Standard Drink?" National Institute on Alcohol Abuse and Alcoholism, https://www.niaaa.nih.gov/alcohols-effects-health/overview-alcohol-consumption/what-standard-drink
Binge drinking for men: "What is Excessive Alcohol Use?" Alcohol and Public Health, https://www.cdc.gov/alcohol/onlinemedia/infographics/excessive-alcohol-use.html
As a CDC infographic emphatically trumpets: ibid
Being intoxicated is acutely unhealthy: "Understanding the Dangers of Alcohol Overdose," National Institute on Alcohol Abuse and Alcoholism, https://www.niaaa.nih.gov/publications/brochures-and-fact-sheets/understanding-dangers-of-alcohol-overdose
half of the deaths and three-quarters of the costs: "Excessive Alcohol Use," National Center for Chronic Disease Prevention and Health Promotion, CDC, https://www.cdc.gov/chronicdisease/resources/publications/factsheets/alcohol.htm
Who binge drinks: "Binge Drinking," CDC, Alcohol and Public Health, https://www.cdc.gov/alcohol/fact-sheets/binge-drinking.htm
higher in people with higher incomes: Dafna Kanny et al., "Annual Total Binge Drinks Consumed by US Adults, 2015," *Am J Prev Med*, April 2018. https://www.ncbi.nlm.nih.gov/pmc/articles/PMC6075714/
consistent across different education levels: Bohm et al., "Binge Drinking Among Adults, by Select Characteristics and State—United States, 2018," *Morbidity and Mortality Weekly Report*, Oct. 2021. https://www.cdc.gov/mmwr/volumes/70/wr/pdfs/mm7041a2-H.pdf
what is now termed alcohol use disorder: "Understanding Alcohol Use Disorder," National Institute on Alcohol Abuse and Alcoholism, NIH, https://www.niaaa.nih.gov/publications/brochures-and-fact-sheets/understanding-alcohol-use-disorder
A 2014 CDC study found that 10%: Marissa Esser et al., "Prevalence of Alcohol Dependence Among US Adult Drinkers, 2009-2011," Preventing Chronic Disease, Public Health Research, Practice, and Policy, CDC. https://www.cdc.gov/pcd/issues/2014/14_0329.htm
Some 10-20% of those who drink excessively: "Alcohol Related Liver Disease," Digestive and Liver Health, University of Michigan Health, https://www.uofmhealth.org/conditions-treatments/digestive-and-liver-health/alcohol-related-liver-disease
a list of situations designed to ferret out: "Diagnostic and Statistical Manual of Mental Disorders (DSM) Alcohol Use Disorder: A Comparison Between DSM-IV and DSM-5," https://www.niaaa.nih.gov/publications/brochures-and-fact-sheets/alcohol-use-disorder-comparison-between-dsm
To replicate this with our diet: Sabine Weiskirchen and Ralf Wesikirchen. "Resveratrol: How Much Wine Do You Have to Drink to Stay Healthy? *Advances in Nutrition*, July 2016. https://www.ncbi.nlm.nih.gov/pmc/articles/PMC4942868/
Caffeine
Rob van Dam et al., "Coffee, Caffeine, and Health," *New England Journal of Medicine*, July 23, 2020, https://www.nejm.org/doi/full/10.1056/NEJMra1816604
has been synthetically derived, not brewed: John Higgins, "Stimulant-Containing Energy Drinks," American College of Cardiology, Feb. 2018. https://www.acc.org/latest-in-cardiology/articles/2018/02/28/10/46/stimulant-containing-ener-

gy-drinks
we tend to overlook the fact: "Spilling the Beans: How Much Caffeine is Too Much?" U.S. FDA,
https://www.fda.gov/consumers/consumer-updates/spilling-beans-how-much-caffeine-too-much
"Although there is no clearly defined threshold…": Aleksandr Voskoboinik et al., "Caffeine and Arrhythmias:
Time to Grind the Data," *J of American College of Cardiology,* April 2018,
https://www.sciencedirect.com/science/article/pii/S2405500X18300756?via%3Dihub
stopping caffeine a minimum of six hours: Christopher Drake, "Caffeine Effects on Sleep Taken 0, 3, or 6
hours before Going to Bed," *Journal of Clinical Sleep Medicine,* Nov 15, 2013 https://jcsm.aasm.org/
doi/10.5664/jcsm.3170

Marijuana
"Marijuana Concentrates DrugFacts," National Institute on Drug Abuse
https://nida.nih.gov/publications/drugfacts/marijuana-concentrates
"Marijuana DrugFacts," National Institute on Drug Abuse
https://nida.nih.gov/publications/drugfacts/marijuana
"Marijuana Research Report," National Institute on Drug Abuse
https://nida.nih.gov/publications/research-reports/marijuana/letter-director
"What You Need to Know (And What We're Working to Find Out) About Products Containing Can-
nabis or Cannabis-derived Compounds, Including CBD," Consumer Updates, U.S. FDA,
https://www.fda.gov/consumers/consumer-updates/what-you-need-know-and-what-were-working-
find-out-about-products-containing-cannabis-or-cannabis
In the early 1990s, average THC levels: "Marijuana Potency," National Institute on Drug Abuse https://
nida.nih.gov/drug-topics/marijuana/marijuana-potency
A 2013-2014 survey: "2013-14 National Roadside Study of Alcohol and Drug Use by Drivers,"
National Highway Traffic Safety Administration, https://www.nhtsa.gov/sites/nhtsa.gov/files/doc-
uments/13013-nrs_drug_092917_v6_tag.pdf
THC use seemed to increase the risk: "Drug and Alcohol Crash Risk Study," p. 4.
National Highway Traffic Safety Administration, https://www.nhtsa.gov/behavioral-research/drug-
and-alcohol-crash-risk-study
A 2017 report from the World Health Organization: "Cannabidiol Pre-Review Report,"
Expert Committee on Drug Dependence, 2017, World Health Organization, https://www.who.int/
medicines/access/controlled-substances/5.2_CBD.pdf

Sleep
"Brain Basics: Understanding Sleep," National Institute of Neurologic Disorders and Stroke,
https://www.ninds.nih.gov/Disorders/patient-caregiver-education/understanding-sleep
Chiara Cirelli and Giulio Tononi, "The Sleeping Brain," *Cerebrum,* May-Jun 2017
https://www.ncbi.nlm.nih.gov/pmc/articles/PMC5501041/
"Healthy Sleep Habits," American Academy of Sleep Medicine, https://sleepeducation.org/healthy-
sleep/healthy-sleep-habits/
"Obstructive Sleep Apnea," American Academy of Sleep Medicine, August 2020, https://sleepedu-
cation.org/sleep-disorders/obstructive-sleep-apnea/#symptoms-of-obstructive-sleep-apnea
"Sleep Health Topics," National Sleep Foundation, https://www.thensf.org/sleep-health-topics/
"What is Insomnia?" American Academy of Sleep Medicine, Sept 2020, https://sleepeducation.org/
sleep-disorders/insomnia/
A consensus statement from the American: Nathaniel Watson et al. "Recommended Amount of Sleep for a
Healthy Adult: A Joint Consensus Statement of the American Academy of Sleep Medicine and Sleep
Research Society," *Sleep,* June 1, 2015, https://www.ncbi.nlm.nih.gov/pmc/articles/PMC4434546/
in 2017, drowsy driving led to: "Drowsy driving," National Highway Safety Administration. https://www.
nhtsa.gov/risky-driving/drowsy-driving
Blue light is a particularly potent suppressor: "Blue light has a dark side," *Harvard Health Publishing,* Harvard

Medical School, July 7, 2020 https://www.health.harvard.edu/staying-healthy/blue-light-has-a-dark-side
everyone's heard of "sleeping pills": "Prescription sleeping pills: What's right for you?" Mayo Clinic, https://www.mayoclinic.org/diseases-conditions/insomnia/in-depth/sleeping-pills/art-20043959
a psychological treatment called: "Cognitive Behavioral Therapy (CBT): Treatment for Insomnia," American Sleep Association, https://www.sleepassociation.org/sleep-treatments/cognitive-behavioral-therapy/

How We Went Cuckoo for Cocoa Puffs
Emily Leib et al. "Nutrition Education for Physicians and Health Professionals: Policy Opportunities for Massachusetts," Food Law and Policy Clinic, Harvard Law School, Sept. 2020, https://chlpi.org/wp-content/uploads/2013/12/MA-Nut-Ed-Issue-Brief-FINALv2.pdf
The Nutrition Source, Harvard T.H. Chan School of Public Health, https://www.hsph.harvard.edu/nutritionsource/
Michael Pollan, *The Omnivore's Dilemma, In Defense of Food, Food Rules,* https://michaelpollan.com/books/
Stephanie Venn-Watson et al. "Efficacy of dietary odd-chain saturated fatty acid pentadeconic acid parallels broad associated health benefits in humans: could it be essential?" *Nature,* May 18, 2020, https://www.nature.com/articles/s41598-020-64960-y
Walter Willett and P.J. Skerrett, *Eat, Drink and Be Healthy: The Harvard Medical School Guide to Healthy Eating,* https://www.hsph.harvard.edu/nutritionsource/2017/10/15/eat-drink-and-be-healthy-willett/
"Give your throat a vacation": Robert Klara, "Throwback Thursday: When Doctors Prescribed 'Healthy' Cigarette Brands," June 2015, *AdWeek,* https://www.adweek.com/brand-marketing/throwback-thursday-when-doctors-prescribed-healthy-cigarette-brands-165404/
"one of the most deleterious cooking oils": Frank Sacks, "Coconut Oil and Heart Health," Jan 2020, *Circulation,* Vol. 141, https://www.ahajournals.org/doi/10.1161/CIRCULATIONAHA.119.044687
FDA declared trans fats to be no longer GRAS: "Trans Fat," US FDA, May 2018. https://www.fda.gov/food/food-additives-petitions/trans-fat
Popular ranch dressing: HiddenValley.com, Nutrition tab https://www.hiddenvalley.com/products/ranch-condiments/original-ranch/original-bottled-ranch/
Then the Prospective Urban Rural Epidemiology (PURE) study: Mahshid Dehghan et al., "Association of fats and carbohydrate intake with cardiovascular disease and mortality in 18 countries from five continents (PURE): a prospective cohort study," *The Lancet,* Nov. 2017, https://www.thelancet.com/article/S0140-6736(17)32252-3/fulltext
A 2016 "Authoritative Review": Dariush Mozaffarian, "Dietary and Policy Priorities for Cardiovascular Disease, Diabetes, and Obesity: A Comprehensive Review," *Circulation,* Jan 12, 2016, https://pubmed.ncbi.nlm.nih.gov/26746178/

Super-Sized Nation
"Adult Body Mass Index," CDC
https://www.cdc.gov/obesity/adult/defining.html
"Adult Overweight & Obesity," CDC
https://www.cdc.gov/obesity/adult/index.html
Dagfinn Aune et al., "BMI and all-cause mortality," *BMJ,* Mar. 2016, https://www.bmj.com/content/353/bmj.i2156
"Diet Reviews," The Nutrition Source, Harvard T.H. Chan School of Public Health
https://www.hsph.harvard.edu/nutritionsource/healthy-weight/diet-reviews/
"Intermittent Fasting: What is it, and how does it work?" Johns Hopkins Medicine
https://www.hopkinsmedicine.org/health/wellness-and-prevention/intermittent-fasting-what-is-it-and-how-does-it-work

We've got a name for it: Metabolic syndrome, Mayo Clinic, https://www.mayoclinic.org/diseases-conditions/metabolic-syndrome/symptoms-causes/syc-20351916

NAFLD is now the most common cause: Bei Li et al, "Nonalcoholic Fatty Liver Disease Cirrhosis: A Review of Its Epidemiology, Risk Factors, Clinical Presentation, Diagnosis, Management, and Prognosis," *Can J Gastroenterology and Hepatology,* July 2018. https://www.ncbi.nlm.nih.gov/pmc/articles/PMC6051295/

the BMI tends to overestimate fat stores: "How good is BMI as an indicator of body fatness?" About Adult BMI, Healthy Weight, Nutrition and Physical Activity, CDC. https://www.cdc.gov/healthyweight/assessing/bmi/adult_bmi/index.html#OtherWays

According to the American Council on Exercise: "Percent Body Fat Norms for Men and Women," Tools and Calculators, *American Council on Exercise,* https://www.acefitness.org/education-and-resources/lifestyle/tools-calculators/percent-body-fat-calculator/

When it comes to fat, sex matters: Kalypso Karastergiou et al., "Sex differences in human adipose tissues—the biology of pear shape," *Biology of Sex Differences,* May 2012. https://www.ncbi.nlm.nih.gov/pmc/articles/PMC3411490/

Research consistently shows that these ketones: Jessica Roekenes and Catia Martins, "A Review: Ketogenic diets and appetite regulation," *Curr Opin Clin Nutr Metab Care,* July 2021. https://pubmed.ncbi.nlm.nih.gov/33883420/

Switching to this fat-burning metabolism: Rafael Cabo and Mark Mattson, "Effects of Intermittent Fasting on Health, Aging, Disease," *New England Journal of Medicine,* Dec. 2019 https://www.nejm.org/doi/full/10.1056/nejmra1905136

an NIH-sponsored study examined: Krista Casazza et al., "Myths, Presumptions, and Facts about Obesity," *New England Journal of Medicine,* Jan. 13, 2013, https://www.ncbi.nlm.nih.gov/pmc/articles/PMC3606061/

Move It or Lose It

"The Benefits of Physical Activity for Brain Health," Physical Activity Guidelines for Americans, 2nd edition; Ch 2, Table 2-3, page 40 https://health.gov/sites/default/files/2019-09/Physical_Activity_Guidelines_2nd_edition.pdf

"Exercise intensity: How to measure it," Healthy Lifestyle Fitness, Mayo Clinic. https://www.mayoclinic.org/healthy-lifestyle/fitness/in-depth/exercise-intensity/art-20046887

"The "NEAT Defect" in Human Obesity: The Role of Nonexercise Activity Thermogenesis," *Mayo Clinic Endocrinology Update,* Vol 2; 1, 2007 https://www.mayoclinic.org/documents/mc5810-0307-pdf/doc-20079082

James A. Levine, "The Chairman's Curse: Lethal Sitting," Mayo Clin Proc., August 2014, https://www.mayoclinicproceedings.org/article/S0025-6196(14)00573-4/pdf

Pedro Villablanca et al., "Nonexercise Activity Thermogenesis in Obesity Management," *Mayo Clinic Proceedings,* 2015. Vol 90 (4), https://www.mayoclinicproceedings.org/article/S0025-6196(15)00123-8/fulltext

"Target Heart Rate and Estimated Maximum Heart Rate," Measuring Physical Activity Intensity, CDC, https://www.cdc.gov/physicalactivity/basics/measuring/heartrate.htm

A sedentary 50-year-old, six-foot: "Adult Energy Needs and BMI Calculator," Baylor College of Medicine, https://www.bcm.edu/cnrc-apps/caloriesneed.cfm

in his book, Move a Little, Lose a Lot: James A. Levine, *Move a Little, Lose a Lot: New N.E.A.T. Science Reveals How to Be Thinner, Happier, and Smarter* https://www.amazon.com/Move-Little-Lose-Lot-T/dp/B005ZOFWTU

In the first study: James Levine et al.; "Role of Nonexercise Activity Thermogenesis in Resistance to Fat Gain in Humans," *Science,* Jan. 199. https://pubmed.ncbi.nlm.nih.gov/9880251/

bacteria in our colon play a role: Claudia Wallis, "How Gut Bacteria Help Make Us Fat and Thin,", *Scientific American,* June 2014, https://www.scientificamerican.com/article/how-gut-bacteria-help-make-

us-fat-and-thin/
Levine did a second study: James Levine et al, "Interindividual variation in posture allocation: possible role in human obesity," *Science,* Jan 2005.
https://pubmed.ncbi.nlm.nih.gov/15681386/
An average Old Order Amish male: David Bassett et al. "Physical activity in an Old Order Amish community," *Med Sci Sports Exerc.* Jan. 2004. https://pubmed.ncbi.nlm.nih.gov/14707772/
"Data collected by devices": "The Relationship Between Sedentary Behavior and Physical Activity," *Physical Activity Guidelines for Americans,* 2nd edition; Ch 1, p. 21
https://health.gov/sites/default/files/2019-09/Physical_Activity_Guidelines_2nd_edition.pdf
A 2011 review out of Duke: Mahesh Patel et al., "Metabolic Deterioration of the Sedentary Control Group in Clinical Trials," *J Appl Physiol,* July 2011, https://journals.physiology.org/doi/pdf/10.1152/japplphysiol.00421.2011
Let me put you inside a graph: "Relationship Among Moderate-to-Vigorous Physical Activity, Sitting Time, and Risk of All-Cause Mortality in Adults," Physical Activity Guidelines for Americans, 2nd edition; Ch 1, Figure 1-3, page 22
https://health.gov/sites/default/files/2019-09/Physical_Activity_Guidelines_2nd_edition.pdf
have the ability to measure telomeres: "What are Telomeres?" News Medical, *Life Sciences*
https://www.news-medical.net/life-sciences/What-are-Telomeres.aspx
researchers studied more than 2,400 pairs: Lynn Cherkas et al., "The Association Between Physical Activity in Leisure Time and Leukocyte Telomere Length," *Archives of Internal Medicine,* Jan. 2008, https://pubmed.ncbi.nlm.nih.gov/18227361/

Rise Up, AARPathletes!
"Exercise and Physical Activity for Older Adults: Position Stand from American College of Sports Medicine," *Medicine & Science in Sport & Exercise,* July 2009, Vol 41 (7). Table 1
https://journals.lww.com/acsm-msse/Fulltext/2009/07000/Exercise_and_Physical_Activity_for_Older_Adults.20.aspx
John Faulkner et al., "The Aging of Elite Male Athletes: age-related changes in performance and skeletal muscle structure function," *Clin J Sports Med;* 2008 Nov; 18 (6): 501-507
https://www.ncbi.nlm.nih.gov/pmc/articles/PMC3928819/
MT Galloway and P Jokl, "Aging Successfully: The Importance of Physical Activity in Maintaining Health and Function," *Journal Am Acad Orthop Surgery,* Jan-Feb 2000; 8 (1):37-44, https://pubmed.ncbi.nlm.nih.gov/10666651/
"2018 Physical Activity Guidelines Advisory Committee Scientific Report," U.S. Department of Health and Human Services https://health.gov/our-work/nutrition-physical-activity/physical-activity-guidelines/current-guidelines/scientific-report
"Physical Activity Guidelines for Americans, 2nd Edition," U.S. Department of Health and Human Services https://health.gov/our-work/nutrition-physical-activity/physical-activity-guidelines/current-guidelines
Scott Trappe, "Master Athletes," *International Journal of Sport Nutrition and Exercise Metabolism;* 2001, Dec., https://pubmed.ncbi.nlm.nih.gov/11915921/
where you land on the infamous "All-Cause Mortality": "Relationship of Moderate-to-Vigorous Physical Activity to All-Cause Mortality," Physical Activity Guidelines for Americans, 2nd edition Ch 2, Fig 2-1, p 35.
https://health.gov/sites/default/files/2019-09/Physical_Activity_Guidelines_2nd_edition.pdf
"The [health] benefits continue to increase": "How Much Total Activity a Week?", Physical Activity Guidelines for Americans, 2nd Edition, Ch 4 p. 57
https://health.gov/our-work/nutrition-physical-activity/physical-activity-guidelines/current-guidelines
Researchers put a small group of men: Lex Verdijk et al., "Skeletal Muscle Hypertrophy Following Resistance Training Is Accompanied by a Fiber Type-Specific Increase in Satellite Cell Content in Elderly Men," *J Gerontol A Biol Sci Med Sci.,* Mar. 2009. https://www.ncbi.nlm.nih.gov/pmc/articles/PMC2655000/

American College of Sports Medicine suggest: "Resistance Training for Health" Infographic, *American College of Sports Medicine* https://www.acsm.org/docs/default-source/files-for-resource-library/resistance-training-for-health.pdf?sfvrsn=d2441c0_2

geek out on this Metabolic Equivalent of Task (MET) stuff: "Compendium of Physical Activities (METs tables)," Arizona State University, Healthy Lifestyles Research Center https://sites.google.com/site/compendiumofphysicalactivities/home?authuser=0

Sexercise

R F Debusk, "Evaluating the Cardiovascular Tolerance for Sex," *American Journal of Cardiology* 2000; 86 (suppl): 51F-56F, https://pubmed.ncbi.nlm.nih.gov/10899280/

A 2007 study in the American Journal of Cardiology: Sebastian Palmeri, et al., "Heart Rate and Blood Pressure Response in Adult Men and Women During Exercise and Sexual Activity," *American Journal of Cardiology*, 2007;100: 1795-1801 https://pubmed.ncbi.nlm.nih.gov/18082530/

"Surrender Dorothy!": "After Hours" (1985). Surrender Dorothy scene. Directed by Martin Scorsese. Written by Joseph Minion, https://www.youtube.com/watch?v=XIRN43cVMHI

A 1984 study managed to do just that: J G Bohlen et al., "Heart Rate, Rate-Pressure Product, and Oxygen Uptake During Four Sexual Activities," *Archives of Internal Medicine*, Vol 144, Sept. 1984 https://pubmed.ncbi.nlm.nih.gov/6476990/

This puts the rigor of sexual activity: "American College of Sports Medicine Guidelines for Exercise Testing and Prescription 10th edition," Table 1.1, Metabolic Equivalents (METs) Values of Common Physical Activities Classified as Light, Moderate, or Vigorous Intensity https://www.acsm.org/docs/default-source/publications-files/acsm-guidelines-download-10th-edabf32a97415a400e9b3be594a6cd-7fbf.pdf?sfvrsn=aaa6d2b2_0

The risk of having a heart attack goes up: J E Muller et al., "Triggering Myocardial Infarction by Sexual Activity," *JAMA*, 1996; 275 (18): 1405-1409, https://pubmed.ncbi.nlm.nih.gov/8618365/

a once-a-week sexcapade: S E Kimmel, "Sex and myocardial infarction: an epidemiologic risk perspective," *Am J Cardiology*, July 20, 2000. https://pubmed.ncbi.nlm.nih.gov/10899270/

anger 3 percent: Robert DeBusk, "Sexual Activity in Patients with Angina," *JAMA*, Dec. 17, 2003, https://jamanetwork.com/journals/jama/article-abstract/197823

Risky Business

So in that spirit, let's take a serious look: "10 Leading Causes of Death, United States; 2019, All Races, Male," WISQARS; National Center for Injury Prevention and Control, Centers for Disease Control and Prevention https://www.cdc.gov/injury/wisqars/pdf/leading_causes_of_death_by_age_group_2018-508.pdf

The heavy hitters in the "unintentional injury" category: "Explore Fatal Injury Data Visualization Tool," WISQARS; National Center for Injury Prevention and Control, Centers for Disease Control and Prevention, https://wisqars.cdc.gov/data/explore-data/home

Eighty percent of spinal cord injuries: "Spinal Cord Injury Fact Sheets," University of Alabama at Birmingham Spinal Cord Injury Model System database https://www.uab.edu/medicine/sci/uab-scims-information/sci-infosheets

"What did I do? I did my job.": The Office, Health Care episode https://theoffice.fandom.com/wiki/Health_Care

Heart Disease

"Coronary Artery Disease," Mayo Clinic, https://www.mayoclinic.org/diseases-conditions/coronary-artery-disease/symptoms-causes/syc-20350613

"Coronary Heart Disease," National Heart, Lung, and Blood Institute, https://www.nhlbi.nih.gov/health-topics/coronary-heart-disease

The primary driver of all forms of atherosclerosis: Göran Hansson, "Inflammation, Atherosclerosis, and Coronary Artery Disease," *New England Journal of Medicine*, April 21, 2005, https://www.nejm.org/doi/full/10.1056/nejmra043430

A 2007 study in the New England Journal of Medicine: William Boden et al., "Optimal Medical Therapy with or without PCI for Stable Coronary Disease," *New England Journal of Medicine*, April 2007. https://www.nejm.org/doi/full/10.1056/nejmoa070829

Dr. Steve Nissen, who at the time: Gardiner Harris, "Doctor Faces Suits Over Cardiac Stents," *New York Times*, Dec 5. 2010 https://www.nytimes.com/2010/12/06/health/06stent.html?pagewanted=all

A seminal 2011 study: Gregg Stone et al., "A Prospective Natural-History Study of Coronary Atherosclerosis," *New England Journal of Medicine*, Nov 2011. https://www.nejm.org/doi/full/10.1056/nejmoa1002358

...delved into what factors were involved: Earl Ford et al., "Explaining the Decrease in U.S. Deaths from Coronary Disease, 1980-2000," *New England Journal of Medicine*, June 7, 2007, https://www.nejm.org/doi/full/10.1056/nejmsa053935

Heart Disease Prevention

"Cardiac CT for Calcium Scoring," RadiologyInfo.org
https://www.radiologyinfo.org/en/info/ct_calscoring

"Diabetes," Mayo Clinic
https://www.mayoclinic.org/diseases-conditions/diabetes/symptoms-causes/syc-20371444

"My Cholesterol Guide," American Heart Association
https://www.heart.org/-/media/Files/Health-Topics/Cholesterol/My-Cholesterol-Guide-English.pdf

Eoin O'Brien et al., "Ambulatory blood pressure monitoring in the 21st century," *Journal of Clinical Hypertension*, July 13, 2018, https://onlinelibrary.wiley.com/doi/full/10.1111/jch.13275

"Blood Pressure Measurement Instructions," American Heart Association https://www.heart.org/-/media/files/health-topics/high-blood-pressure/how_to_measure_your_blood_pressure_letter_size.pdf

The study found that nine risk factors: Salim Yusuf et al., "Effect of potentially modifiable risk factors associated with myocardial infarction in 52 countries (the INTERHEART study): case-control study," *The Lancet*, Sept. 11, 2004, https://www.thelancet.com/journals/lancet/article/PIIS0140-6736(04)17018-9/fulltext

I'll suggest you go online and find: American College of Cardiology Risk Estimator Plus https://tools.acc.org/ascvd-risk-estimator-plus/#!/calculate/estimate/

That's a big deal because according to the 2018 American Heart Association: Scott Grundy et al. "2.4, Monitoring Response of LDL-C to Statin Therapy," 2018 AHA/ACC Guideline on the Management of Blood Cholesterol, *Circulation*, Nov 2018. https://www.ahajournals.org/doi/10.1161/cir.0000000000000625#d3e1518

According to the CDC, 116 million: "High Blood Pressure," CDC https://www.cdc.gov/bloodpressure/facts.htm

ABPM has shown us what we're missing: Eoin O'Brien et al., "Ambulatory Blood Pressure Measurement: What is the International Consensus?" *Hypertension*, Sept. 2013. https://www.ahajournals.org/doi/full/10.1161/hypertensionaha.113.02148

for individual patients at low risk, the benefits of a daily aspirin: "Aspirin Use to Prevent Cardiovascular Disease and Colorectal Cancer: Preventive Medication," U.S. Preventive Services Task Force, https://www.uspreventiveservicestaskforce.org/uspstf/recommendation/aspirin-to-prevent-cardiovascular-disease-and-cancer

Cancer, the Big "C"

"Cancer diagnosis and staging," National Cancer Institute,
https://www.cancer.gov/about-cancer/diagnosis-staging/diagnosis

"Cancer Screening Overview—Patient Version," National Cancer Institute

https://www.cancer.gov/about-cancer/screening/patient-screening-overview-pdq
"Crunching Numbers: What Cancer Screening Statistics Really Tell Us," National Cancer Institute,
https://www.cancer.gov/about-cancer/screening/research/what-screening-statistics-mean
"HPV-associated cancers," HPV and Cancer, CDC
https://www.cdc.gov/cancer/hpv/statistics/index.htm
"Risk Factors for Cancer," Cancer Causes and Prevention, About Cancer, National Cancer Institute,
https://www.cancer.gov/about-cancer/causes-prevention/risk
"Types of Cancer Treatment," National Cancer Institute
https://www.cancer.gov/about-cancer/treatment/types
"Targeted therapy to treat cancer," "Immunotherapy to treat cancer,"
https://www.cancer.gov/about-cancer/treatment/types/targeted-therapies
https://www.cancer.gov/about-cancer/treatment/types/immunotherapy
A report from the National Research Council calculated: David Spiegelhalter, "How likely am I to be hit by an asteroid?" BBC Future, Feb 22, 2012 https://www.bbc.com/future/article/20120222-waiting-for-a-rock-to-fall
Cancer and heart disease jockey: "Top 10 Cancers by Rates of New Cancer Cases, 2018," "Top 10 Cancers by Rates of Cancer Deaths, 2018," United States Cancer Statistics: Data Visualizations, CDC https://gis.cdc.gov/Cancer/USCS/#/AtAGlance/
wrinkles in the racial demographics of cancer: "Cancer Statistics At a Glance, New Cases or Deaths," United States Cancer Statistics: Data Visualizations, CDC. Use "Race and Ethnicity" tab.
https://gis.cdc.gov/Cancer/USCS/#/AtAGlance/
It is not typically one single mutation: Siddhartha Mukherjee, *The Emperor of All Maladies.* A biography of cancer, https://www.amazon.com/Emperor-All-Maladies-Biography-Cancer/dp/1439170916
"These recommendations [for less routine screening]": Cancer Prevention Overview—Patient Version, National Cancer Institute https://www.cancer.gov/about-cancer/causes-prevention/patient-prevention-overview-pdq#section/all
Smoking caused the premature death of 100 million: World Health Organization Report on the Global Tobacco Epidemic, 2008 https://apps.who.int/iris/handle/10665/43818
But the good news is that the body can forgive: Prabhat Jha et al., "21st-Century Hazards of Smoking and Benefits of Cessation in the United States," *New England Journal of Medicine,* Jan 2013, https://www.nejm.org/doi/full/10.1056/NEJMsa1211128#t=articleTop
You can avoid skin cancer: "Sun Exposure & Skin Cancer," Cleveland Clinic, https://my.clevelandclinic.org/health/diseases/10985-sun-exposure-and-skin-cancer
Vaccination could prevent more than 90%: "Cancers Caused by HPV are Preventable," Human Papilloma Virus (HPV), CDC, https://www.cdc.gov/hpv/hcp/protecting-patients.html
"Our bodies, our cells, our genes are thus": Siddhartha Mukherjee, *The Emperor of All Maladies.* A biography of cancer. P. 446.
https://www.amazon.com/Emperor-All-Maladies-Biography-Cancer/dp/1439170916
That new car smell: Nick Kurczewski, "The Science of the New-Car Smell," *Car and Driver,* Jul. 2021, https://www.architecturaldigest.com/story/what-is-off-gassing
a comprehensive list of known or likely: "The Pollution in People: Cancer-Causing Chemicals in Americans' Bodies," Environmental Working Group, June 14, 2016. https://www.ewg.org/research/pollution-people

Lung Cancer

"Lung Cancer," Medical Knowledge Self-Assessment Program® (MKSAP) 18, American College of Physicians.
"Lung Cancer: Early Detection, Diagnosis, and Staging," American Cancer Society
https://www.cancer.org/cancer/lung-cancer/detection-diagnosis-staging.html
"Lung Cancer Prevention," National Cancer Institute

https://www.cancer.gov/types/lung/hp/lung-prevention-pdq#_206_toc
"National Lung Screening Trial," National Cancer Institute
https://www.cancer.gov/types/lung/research/nlst
"Non-Small Cell Lung Cancer Treatment—Patient Version," National Cancer Institute
https://www.cancer.gov/types/lung/patient/non-small-cell-lung-treatment-pdq
"Small Cell Lung Cancer Treatment—Patient Version," National Cancer Institute
https://www.cancer.gov/types/lung/patient/small-cell-lung-treatment-pdq
"Who Should Be Screened for Lung Cancer?" CDC, Lung Cancer
https://www.cdc.gov/cancer/lung/basic_info/screening.htm

Colorectal Cancer
"Colorectal Cancer," Medical Knowledge Self-Assessment Program® (MKSAP) 18, American College of Physicians.
"Colorectal Cancer: Early Detection, Diagnosis, and Staging," American Cancer Society
https://www.cancer.org/cancer/colon-rectal-cancer/detection-diagnosis-staging.html
"Colon Cancer Treatment—Patient version," National Cancer Institute
https://www.cancer.gov/types/colorectal/patient/colon-treatment-pdq
"Rectal Cancer Treatment—Patient Version," National Cancer Institute
https://www.cancer.gov/types/colorectal/patient/rectal-treatment-pdq
"Colorectal Cancer Screening—Patient Version," National Cancer Institute
https://www.cancer.gov/types/colorectal/patient/colorectal-screening-pdq
"Colon Pathology: Understanding Your Pathology Report," American Cancer Society
https://www.cancer.org/treatment/understanding-your-diagnosis/tests/understanding-your-pathology-report/colon-pathology.html
"Colorectal Cancer Prevention—Patient Version," National Cancer Institute
https://www.cancer.gov/types/colorectal/patient/colorectal-prevention-pdq
"Cruciferous Vegetables and Cancer Prevention," National Cancer Institute
https://www.cancer.gov/about-cancer/causes-prevention/risk/diet/cruciferous-vegetables-fact-sheet
A CDC report noted that in 2018: Djenaba Joseph et al., "Vital Signs: Colorectal Cancer Screening Test Use—United States, 2018," MMWR, CDC, March 2020
https://www.cdc.gov/mmwr/volumes/69/wr/mm6910a1.htm
That information, coupled with a 15 percent: Karina Davidson et al., "Screening for Colorectal Cancer, US Preventive Services Task Force Recommendation Statement," *JAMA*, May 2021
https://jamanetwork.com/journals/jama/articlepdf/2779985/jama_davidson_2021_us_210011_1629739999.39667.pdf

Prostate Cancer
Katy Bell et al., "Prevalence of incidental prostate cancer: a systematic review of autopsy studies," Int J Cancer, Oct 1, 2015, https://pubmed.ncbi.nlm.nih.gov/25821151/
"Evidence Summary, Prostate Cancer: Screening," US Preventive Services Task Force
https://www.uspreventiveservicestaskforce.org/uspstf/document/evidence-summary/prostate-cancer-screening#tab3
"Is Prostate Cancer Screening Right for You?" US Preventive Services Task Force,
https://www.documentcloud.org/documents/3549521-Prostate-screening-understanding-risks-and.html
"Prostate Cancer," Medical Knowledge Self-Assessment Program® (MKSAP) 18, American College of Physicians.
"Prostate Cancer Prevention—Health Professional Version," "Risk Factors for Prostate Cancer Development," National Cancer Institute

https://www.cancer.gov/types/prostate/hp/prostate-prevention-pdq# 79
"Prostate Cancer Screening—Patient Version," National Cancer Institute
https://www.cancer.gov/types/prostate/patient/prostate-screening-pdq
"Prostate Cancer Treatment—Patient version," National Cancer Institute
https://www.cancer.gov/types/prostate/patient/prostate-treatment-pdq
"Prostate-Specific Antigen (PSA) Test," National Cancer Institute
https://www.cancer.gov/types/prostate/psa-fact-sheet
"Understanding Your Pathology Report: Prostate Cancer," American Cancer Society
https://www.cancer.org/treatment/understanding-your-diagnosis/tests/understanding-your-pathology-report/prostate-pathology/prostate-cancer-pathology.html
microscopic amounts of prostate cancer in 27 percent: W A Sakr et al., "The Frequency of Carcinoma and Intraepithelial Neoplasia of the Prostate in Young Male Patients," *Journal of Urology*, Aug 1993, https://www.auajournals.org/doi/abs/10.1016/S0022-5347%2817%2935487-3
autopsy study on men who died after age 60: W A Sakr et al., "Age and racial distribution of prostatic intraepithelial neoplasia," *Eur Urol*, 1996;30:138-144. https://pubmed.ncbi.nlm.nih.gov/8875194/
As an article in the New England Journal of Medicine put it: H Gilbert Welch and Peter Albertsen, "Reconsidering Prostate Cancer Mortality—The Future of PSA Screening," *New England Journal of Medicine*, April 16, 2020, https://www.nejm.org/doi/full/10.1056/NEJMms1914228
Even so, two years after surgery: "Prostate Cancer, Treatment," Medical Knowledge Self-Assessment Program® (MKSAP) 18, American College of Physicians, p. 90.
the risk of erectile dysfunction is perhaps: ibid
In 2018, the U.S. Preventive Services Task Force: "Screening for Prostate Cancer: US Preventive Services Task Force Recommendation Statement," *JAMA*, May 2018; 319 (18) https://jamanetwork.com/journals/jama/fullarticle/2680553
at 13 years of follow-up: Fritz Schröder et al., "Screening and prostate cancer mortality: results of the European Randomised Study of Screening for Prostate Cancer (ERSPC) at 13 years of follow-up," *Lancet*, Dec 2014, https://pubmed.ncbi.nlm.nih.gov/25108889/
If one screened 1,000 men: "Is Prostate Cancer Screening Right for You?" graphic, US Preventive Services Task Force, https://www.documentcloud.org/documents/3549521-Prostate-screening-understanding-risks-and.html
If one screened 1,000 men: "Table. Estimated Effects After 13 Years of Inviting Men Aged 55 to 69 Years in the United States to PSA-Based Screening for Prostate Cancer," Final Recommendation Statement, Prostate Cancer: Screening, USPSTF, May 2018. https://www.uspreventiveservicestaskforce.org/uspstf/document/RecommendationStatementFinal/prostate-cancer-screening#bootstrap-panel--10
ERSPC published more encouraging follow-up data: Jonas Hugosson et al., "A 16-year follow-up of the European Randomized study of Screening for Prostate Cancer," *Eur Urol*, July 2019. https://pubmed.ncbi.nlm.nih.gov/30824296/
A 2020 piece in the New England Journal of Medicine: H Gilbert Welch and Peter Albertsen, "Reconsidering Prostate Cancer Mortality—The Future of PSA Screening," *New England Journal of Medicine*, April 16, 2020, https://www.nejm.org/doi/full/10.1056/NEJMms1914228

Mind Games
R H Belemaker and Galila Agam, "Major Depressive Disorder," New England Journal of Medicine, Jan. 3, 2008, https://www.nejm.org/doi/10.1056/NEJMra073096
"The Diagnostic and Statistical Manual of Mental Disorders-5 (DSM-5-TR)," American Psychiatry Association, https://www.psychiatry.org/psychiatrists/practice/dsm
"Mental Health Conditions," National Alliance on Mental Illness (NAMI) https://nami.org/About-Mental-Illness/Mental-Health-Conditions
"Mental Health Information," National Institute of Mental Health https://www.nimh.nih.gov/health/topics

Gayatri Patel et al., "Generalized Anxiety Disorder," *Annals of Internal Medicine*, Dec. 3, 2013, https://www.acpjournals.org/doi/full/10.7326/0003-4819-159-11-201312030-01006

"SAMHSA's (Substance Abuse and Mental Health Services Administration) National Helpline," 1-800-662-HELP (4357), or Samhsa.gov
https://www.samhsa.gov/find-help/national-helpline

"What are Anxiety Disorders?" American Psychiatric Association, https://www.psychiatry.org/patients-families/anxiety-disorders/what-are-anxiety-disorders

"What is Depression?" American Psychiatric Association, https://www.psychiatry.org/patients-families/depression/what-is-depression

According to the National Alliance on Mental Illness: "Mental Health Facts in America, National Alliance on Mental Illness, https://www.nami.org/nami/media/nami-media/infographics/generalmhfacts.pdf

suicide rates have increased 35% since 1999: Anne Case and Angus Deaton, "Mortality and Morbidity in the 21st Century," Brookings Papers on Economic Activity, Spring 2017
https://www.brookings.edu/bpea-articles/mortality-and-morbidity-in-the-21st-century/

The largest increases were noted: Joel Achenbach and Dan Keating, "New Research Identifies a 'Sea of Despair' Among White, Working-Class Americans," *Washington Post*, March 23, 2017,
https://www.washingtonpost.com/national/health-science/new-research-identifies-a-sea-of-despair-among-white-working-class-americans/2017/03/22/c777ab6e-0da6-11e7-9b0d-d27c98455440_story.html

You're Going to Live Forever

"Biology of Aging, Recent Advances," National Institute on Aging
https://www.nia.nih.gov/about/budget/biology-aging-3

"Biology of Aging: Research Today for a Healthier Tomorrow," National Institute on Aging (NIH, U.S. Dept. of Health and Human Services), Pub. No. 11-7561, Nov. 2011
https://storage.googleapis.com/edcompass/quantum/materials/2158_biology_of_aging.pdf

James Fries, "Aging, Natural Death, and the Compression of Morbidity," *New England Journal of Medicine*, July 1980; 303. https://www.ncbi.nlm.nih.gov/pmc/articles/PMC2567746/pdf/11984612.pdf

The human genome consists of 23 pairs: "What is a genome?" Human Genome Project FAQ, National Human Genome Research Institute, https://www.genome.gov/human-genome-project/Completion-FAQ

Mammals, for instance, get about a billion: "The Heart Project, Beats per Life graph" NC State, The Public Science Lab http://robdunnlab.com/projects/beats-per-life/

a life expectancy that may reach into the 70's: "Species Directory, Gray Whale," National Oceanic and Atmospheric Administration. https://www.fisheries.noaa.gov/species/gray-whale

...get closer to 2.5 billion heartbeats: Nova, Amazing Heart Facts
https://www.pbs.org/wgbh/nova/heart/heartfacts.html

Life expectancy in the U.S. in 1900: James Fries, "Aging, Natural Death, and the Compression of Morbidity," *New England Journal of Medicine*, July 1980; Vol.303. Fig. 1
https://www.ncbi.nlm.nih.gov/pmc/articles/PMC2567746/pdf/11984612.pdf

He's spent his career studying: Dan Buettner, "Blue Zones® Power 9®, Reverse Engineering Longevity,"
https://www.bluezones.com/2016/11/power-9/#

Reliable Sources

As all of us have experienced, searching the internet for information can lead one to some strange places, and that holds true for medical information. Website development has become so cheap and sophisticated that a webpage from the prestigious *New England Journal of Medicine* can carry the same visual authority as someone selling probiotics out of a storage unit in San Bernadino.

So, I recommend sticking with the tried and true, the reliable and trustworthy. Here are a few suggestions:

The Centers for Disease Control and Prevention (CDC).
https://www.cdc.gov/

The National Institutes of Health (NIH) is part of the U.S. Department of Health and Human Services. It's a collection of 27 Institutes and Centers, each with its own particular health focus. You saw the National Cancer Institute, National Institute of Drug Abuse, National Institute of Mental Health and others on my endnotes list above.
https://www.nih.gov/

MedlinePlus: a service of the National Library of Medicine. I particularly like its drug information.
https://medlineplus.gov/

U.S. Food & Drug Administration
https://www.fda.gov/

World Health Organization
https://www.who.int/

Large healthcare systems like Mayo Clinic, Johns Hopkins Medicine, Cleveland Clinic, Harvard Medical School, Kaiser Permanente etc. are reliable sources for health information (click here now to schedule an appointment with one of our providers), as are well-recognized disease-focused organizations like the American Lung Association, National Alliance on Mental Illness, American Cancer Society, and American Heart Association.

If you're looking for information on nutrition, tread lightly on diet plan websites that want to sell you something. Instead, take a look at "The Nutrition Source" website at Harvard's T.H. Chan School of Public Health. One of their lead professors, Walter C. Willett, is arguably the world's most knowledgeable nutritionist, and his best-selling book *Eat, Drink, and Be Healthy* masterfully brings the bench science of nutrition to the kitchen counter.